POPULAR LECTURES IN

Undergraduate Mathematics

POPULAR LECTURES IN

Undergraduate Mathematics

SADASHIV G DEO
DAMODAR Y KASTURE
H V KUMBHOJKAR
VASANT G TIKEKAR

Universities Press

UNIVERSITIES PRESS (INDIA) PRIVATE LIMITED

Registered Office
3-6-747/1/A & 3-6-754/1, Himayatnagar,
Hyderabad 500 029 (A.P.), India
e-mail: info@universitiespress.com

Distributed by
Orient Blackswan Private Limited

Registered Office
3-6-752 Himayatnagar, Hyderabad 500 029 (A.P.) India

Other Offices
Bangalore / Bhopal / Bhubaneshwar / Chennai
Ernakulam / Guwahati / Hyderabad / Jaipur / Kolkata
Lucknow / Mumbai / New Delhi / Patna

First published 2009

ISBN 978 81 7371 662 1

Typeset in Book Antiqua 10.5/12.6 by
Techastra Solutions (P) Ltd,
Hyderabad 500 029

Printed in India by
Orion Printers Private Limited
Hyderabad 500 004

Published by
Universities Press (India) Private Limited
3-6-747/1/A & 3-6-754/1, Himayatnagar,
Hyderabad 500 029 (A.P.), India

Dedicated to our beloved respected teachers

Prof V Lakshmikantham

Professor, Florida Institute of Technology Melbourne (FL), USA

Prof S D Nigam

Ex. Professor, IIT, Chennai

Prof Krishna Tewari

Ex. Professor, IIT, Kanpur

Late Prof P L Bhatnagar

Ex. Professor, IISc., Bangalore

Contents

Preface

"Mathematics is a way of thinking which enables students to see unifying patterns in diverse context" said an inspired teacher of mathematics to a class room full of college students. The entire class was blank – you could almost see the question mark on each face. The statement made by the teacher is true but the students did not have the knowledge background to appreciate such a lofty remark. Their learning process was restricted to a textbook, to few chapters in it, defined by the syllabi. Never in their life were they posed questions like, "What is mathematics? What mathematics should we learn and why? What does it have to do with real life? How much mathematics should one learn?", nor have their teachers attempted to raise these questions and answer them. The sad conclusion that we must face is that there is a lacuna in our learning process.

Most students have a very limited view of mathematical literature since they progress through a narrow path of textbooks. At the end of their career they find that they know only a few things about this vast field which is their specialisation. For example, a question was asked in an examination paper: What is the next term in the sequence $\{2, 4, 6, 8, \cdots\}$? Most answered that it was 10. It was only after reading an article, that they realised that their answer was only partial. In fact, the question posed itself is incorrect. Very few students know that there are several geometries other than Euclidean, or that there are several problems in mathematics which remain unsolved. Most students do not know that the subject of mathematics has an important role in biological, medical, social sciences, modern technologies as also in aesthetics. While pointing out these shortcomings, we do not blame anyone. It is only an objective observation. One must find a solution to reduce the gap in our teaching and learning process in mathematics education.

One of the solutions is complementing the learning process by self-learning devices and popular-general lecturing schemes by experts in the field. Further, our teachers need to be alert, abreast with breakthroughs in the field and provide exact definitions of new concepts. They must carefully draft the proofs of various theorems, and mention limitations, provide suitably designed examples and counter-examples and continuously evaluate the outcome of the teaching process. Further, when need arises, the instructor must remove the parallax between teaching and learning. For enhancing the confidence of students in mathematics, they must receive clear answers to the questions like those raised here in the first paragraph. Quite often a well-written textbook also needs augumentation with additional information. Once a student is convinced about the spirit of the subject of his choice, its strengths and limitations, its history and future, its relations with real-life situations, its beauty and intellectual challenges, he/she generally becomes a candidate for advanced courses in mathematics. The learning process for him is then a fountain of delight and pleasure.

The aim of the present book is to provide a modest approach along this path of teaching and learning. The authors were invited by many universities, colleges, seminars and conferences to deliver the lectures on the topics presented in the following pages and many others which could not be included here because of limitations of space. We sincerely feel that through these lectures, the gap between class-room teaching and learning was reduced. Students found their confidence boosted with the realisation of the strength of their subject of choice.

All the authors are closely associated with the Marathwada Mathematical Society, Aurangabad. Their aim is to emphasise teaching of mathematics at the undergraduate and postgraduate level. Their objectives were at the core when the authors took the decision to write this book.

The present volume includes well-selected popular lectures which clearly brings together the answers to the questions posed at the beginning of this preface. The lectures are written so that the student does not require a teacher. They can discover by themselves that there are answers in the present book which clear their doubts. The language and flow of the contents are carefully structured so as to make the writing students-friendly. The text of the book takes into account the level and age group of the undergraduate students. Teachers of mathematics may find some of these lectures of immediate use to make their classroom work more innovative, promising and fruitful. The amateur mathematician may also find something new in its modernity, application orientation and creativity. The book also provides scope for students and teachers to formulate some interesting mathematical projects for their curriculum requirements.

The innovative lecture series included in the following pages consists of the following areas.

The first lecture provides information on the Fields Medals, the highest award in mathematics, considered equivalent to the Nobel Prize. A list of award winners and their specialisations are included. Lectures 2, 3 and 4 speak about the philosophy and logic of mathematics and its historical perspective. Lectures 5 and 6 present the spirit of mathematics as a discipline.

Lecture 7 leads to reality and its relation with mathematics through the concept of fuzzy logic. Conjectures in mathematics have been a source of constant challenge to the human brain. Some of them are solved, while many remain unsolved. This forms the subject matter of Lecture 8. Teaching and learning processes are described in Lecture 9. Lectures 10 and 11 speak about numbers, while Lecture 12 includes various facts of an elementary diagram—the triangle. The important problem of detecting and correcting errors in transmitted messages through computers is solved in Lecture 13 using elementary group theory. The concept of "distance" from modern analysis is the subject of Lecture 14.

Differential equation methods form a part of applied mathematics. Lectures 15, 16, 17 and 18 provide applications of these methods in modelling extended trigonometry. Lecture 18 focusses on the decision process while Lectures 19 to 22 include applications to modern technologies and social sciences.

Any book, however big, cannot do justice to the total spread of mathematical topics. However, some mile-stones provided through these lectures bring out the essence of mathematics' reach. Students, once they focus their efforts, can progress through self-learning programmes to other topics which interest them. With this purpose in mind, the authors have provided an exhaustive bibliography and suggested additional literature. It is possible for teachers to use this book while preparing projects for students as a part of the curriculum compliance.

On the Indian scene, there are yet not many books of this kind. The authors hope that the present work will fill this gap and that the teachers and students benefit from its reading.

There are many individuals whose valuable help made it possible to prepare the present manuscript and finally get it published.

Dr Gopal R Shendge and Dr Sudhakar R Joshi from Aurangabad, Dr Sree Hari Rao from Hyderabad, made useful suggestions to improve the contents. The authors express their sincere gratitude to them for their untiring efforts. The typesetting of the original manuscript was done by Shri Nitin Mahindrakar of PageMaker, and Mr. Balwant Mahajan both from Aurangabad. Their help made it possible to get the manuscript ready on time. We record our sincere thanks to them. Further, we take pleasure in thanking Shri. Madhu Reddy, Universities Press (India) Pvt. Ltd. Hyderabad, and his colleagues for their efforts in publishing this book in its present form.

March, 2009

Panaji, Goa.

Lecture 1

History of the Fields Medals

Abstract

The present lecture takes us through the inception of the Nobel prizes and speculates why there is no Nobel prize in mathematics. This is followed by a brief history of the Fields Medals ending with a list of the recipients since it was first awarded in 1936.

1.1 Introduction

Alfred Bernhard Nobel (1833–1896) is more known for his philanthropic nature and the prize that was named after him than his contributions as a chemical scientist. Nobel trained in chemical engineering and was the inventor of dynamite. This safe form of nitroglycerine was soon put to use in blasting tunnels, cutting canals, and building railways and roads. Nobel amassed a great fortune with his patent. Although his inventions were central to destruction and the art of making war, Nobel loved peace. He also derived pleasure from literature and as an inventor, believed in the promotion of science as a way of uplifting humanity. In his will he set aside a substantial amount of his estate to establish yearly awards for the greatest contributions in physics, chemistry, medicine, literature and world peace. The Nobel awards have been presented since 1901. In 1969, a Nobel prize for economics was also instituted.

Alfred considered mathematics the queen of sciences. Knowing this, it has been a source of constant curiosity, why he did not include an award for mathematics. One of the most common yet unverified reasons stated is his antipathy towards M G Mittag-Leffeler (1848–1927). The story goes that if a Nobel prize for mathematics had been instituted,

Mittag-Leffeler would have been a prime candidate for it, because of his important discoveries in mathematics – this was not something Nobel, with his personal grudge against him, would have liked.

Interesting though this might be, the more likely reason would be that the prizes were awarded for those "inventions or discoveries" of greatest practical benefit to mankind. Mathematics, considered a theoretical subject at that time, might not have fit in this criteria – even now the physics prize is awarded more for experimental work than for advances in theory.

During the last century, the prize has grown in importance to become the most prestigious in the world. It has in some ways spurred scientists on to higher and higher levels of knowledge in the search for the holy grail.

1.2 John Charles Fields

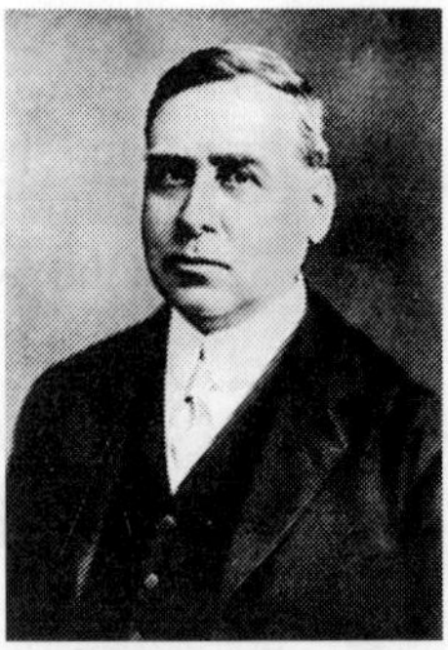

It was John Charles Fields (1863–1932) who seriously thought of filling the gap left by Alfred Nobel. Fields was born in Hamilton (in Ontorio, Canada). He graduated from the University of Toronto, Canada in 1884 and got his doctorate (1887) from the John Hopkins University in USA. This university is known – even today – as one of the great institutions for original research. He spent 10 years in Europe and worked with several leading mathematicians of that time. He returned to Canada in 1902 and was elected fellow of the Royal Society of Canada and the Royal Society of London. He also played a leading role in the Royal Canadian Institution and was its president between 1919 to 1925. Although Fields did his thesis on differential equations, he later published several papers in algebraic functions.

In 1924, Fields was a chairperson of the International Congress of Mathematicians (ICM) held at Toronto, Canada. He felt that there should be a prize, equivalent to a Nobel award, for mathematics so that an outstanding mathematician will be honoured for his distinguished contributions. During the proceedings of the ICM he saved \$2700 – a sizable sum in those days. He proposed that out of this money two medals be presented to young mathematicians on the occasion of ICM gatherings in the future.

1.3 History

In 1932, a committee charted out the process of selecting outstanding mathematicians. It was decided that the award should recognise the merit of the winner, yet it should provide enough boost to help him in his pursuit of future discoveries. Further, it should stimulate others to compete for the prize. Hence it was decided that the awards should be made to a young mathematician below the age of 40 years who has broken the barriers of earlier achievements and opened new areas of discoveries. Thus these medals were not meant as a recognition of the life-time achievements of senior mathematicians. It was further decided that these awards be presented at the International Congress of Mathematicians (ICM) meeting scheduled for September 1932 at Zurich. It was indeed unfortunate that shortly before this meeting, Prof. John Fields expired and the awards could not be made. However before his death, Fields had decided the nature of the medals and the inscriptions on both its sides. The face side of the medal consists of a picture of the Greek mathematician Archimedes (287–212 BCE). The Latin inscription around it reads: " To transcend one's human limitations and master the universe ". The other side of the medal consists of a Latin inscription which reads " Mathematicians gathered together from the whole world honour the noteworthy contributions to knowledge. " There is also carved, on the background, an Archimedes sphere inscribed in a cylinder. The name of the recipient of the award is engraved on the rim of the medal. Prof. Fields even decided the size of these medals—7.5 centimeters in diameter, made of pure gold.

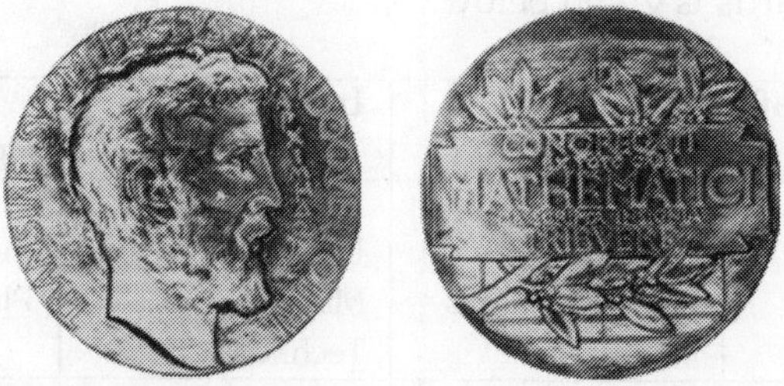

In 1934, the National Trust Company in Canada was appointed the Chief Trustee of the prize fund. Prof. Fields had also left some money in his will for the purpose of these awards. The medal was finally designed by a well-known sculptor of Canada, Dr. R T McKenzie. The medal together with a cash award is presented to the outstanding mathematician.

A curious reader might ask, how are mathematicians selected for the award? Mathematics is such a vast subject, rapidly developing in different areas. Further, now several countries have proved that they possess mathematical talent worth the name. Naturally, selection of the right person is a complex issue.

The ICM meeting is held every four years and attended by thousands of scientists. The ICM appoints an international committee of experts (7–8 members). This committee prepares a list of 30 candidates who have made important path-breaking contributions. Further eliminations are made and thorough discussions spread over a period of two years, a final list of two to four mathematicians is approved. As the age of the awardee is restricted to 40 years, there are cases when outstanding mathematicians who succeed in resolving complex mathematical problems miss the chance of getting the Fields Medal – only because they are over the age of 40.

The first ever Fields Medals were awarded to two mathematicians in 1936 at the ICM meeting held at Oslo. Because of the Second World War, ICM meetings were not held for 14 years. It was only in 1950 that an ICM meeting was held again in Cambridge, Massachusetts (USA) when two medals were awarded. Since then Fields Medals have been awarded to two to four mathematicians every four years.

1.4 The Awardees

The most recent ICM meeting was held at Madrid, Spain between August 22–30, 2006. It takes 7–8 years of preparations to organise such a gigantic conference. The next ICM meeting in the year 2010 will be held in India. So far, no Indian mathematician has received this award, although Indians have been members of the selection committees in the past. A table of the recipients of the Fields Medals, their specialisation, their institutions and the year of awards is given below.

Year/Place of ICM	Recipients	Institution	Area of Specialisation
1936 Oslo	1. L V Alfors	Harvard University	Complex function theory
	2. Jesse Douglas	Mass. Inst. of Tech. USA	Plateau problem
1950	1. L Schwartz	Univ. of Nancy, France	Theory of distributions
Cambridge Massachusetts	2. A Selberg	Institute for Advanced Studies, USA	Number theory
1954	1. K Kodaira	Princeton University	Deformation of structures and theory of surfaces

Year/Place of ICM	Recipients	Institution	Area of Specialisation
Amsterdam	2. J P Serre	University of Paris	Algebraic topology
1958 Edinburgh	1. K F Roth	University of London	Number theory
	2. René Thom	Universtiy of Strasbourg, France	Differential topology
1962 Edinburgh	1. L H Hörmander	University of Stockholm	Differential equations
	2. J W Milnor	Princeton University	Topology
1966 Moscow	1. M F Atiyah	Oxford University	Differential operators and geometry
	2. P J Cohen	Stanford University	Logic and set theory
	3. A Grothendieck	University of Paris	Algebraic geometry
	4. S Smale	University of California	Differential topology
1970 Nice, France	1. A Baker	Cambridge University	Number theory
	2. H Hironaka	Harvard University	Algebraic geometry (study of singularities)
	3. S P Novikov	Moscow University	Topology
	4. J G Thompson	Cambridge University	Group theory
1974 Vancouver	1. E Bombieri	University of Pisa	Number theory and geometry
	2. D Mumford	Harvard University	Algebraic geometry (Moduli problems)
1978 Helesinki	1. P Deligne	IHES, France	Algebraic geometry and number theory
	2. C Fefferman	Princeton University	Classic analysis and differential equations

Year/Place of ICM	Recipients	Institution	Area of Specialisation
	3. G A Margulis	Institute for Problems in Information Transmission, Moscow	Discrete subgroups of Lie groups
	4. D Quillen	Massachusetts Institute of Technology	Topology and K-theory
1982 Warsaw	1. A Connes	Center National La Rech Scientifique, France	Differential geometry
	2. W B Thurston	Princeton University	Topology
	3. S T Yau	Harvard University	Partial differential equations and algebraic geometry
1986 Berkeley	1. S Donaldson	University of Oxford	Four dimensions of geometry
	2. G Faltings	Princeton University	Algebraic geometry
	3. M Freedman	University of California at San Diago	Poincare conjecture
1990 Kyoto	1. V Drinfeld	Academy of SCS of Ukraine	Quantum theory
	2. V Jones	University of California at Berkeley	Neumann algebra and geometric topology
	3. S Mori	Kyoto Univeristy, Japan	Algebraic geometry
	4. E Witten	Institute for Advanced Studies at Princeton	Differential geometry
1994 Zurich	1. P L Lions	University of Paris	Nonlinear partial differential Equations
	2. J C Yoccoz	University of Paris	Dynamical systems
	3. J Bourgain	University of Illinois	Mathematical analysis
	4. E Zelmanov	University of Chicago	Nilpotent groups

Year/Place of ICM	Recipients	Institution	Area of Specialisation
1998 Montreal	1. R E Borcherds	Cambridge University	Atmospheric forms and mathematical physics
	2. W T Gowers	Cambridge University	Functional analysis and combinatorics
	3. M Kontsevich	IHES, France and Rutgers University, USA	Algebraic geometry, algebraic topology, and mathematical physics
	4. C T McMullen	Harvard University	Holomorphic dynamics, geometry of 3-dimensional manifolds
2002 Beijing	1. Laurent Lafforgue	IHES, France	Langland's programme (number theory and analysis)
	2. Valdimir Voevodsky	Institute of Advanced Studies at Princeton University	Algebraic varieties (number and algebraic geometry)
2006 Madrid	1. Andrei Okounkov	Princeton University	Bridging probability, representation theory and algebraic geometry
	2. Terence Tau	University of California Los Angeles	Prime numbers
	3. Wendelin Werner	University of Paris	Probability theory and mathematical physics

In 1981, the International Mathematical Union (IMU) established the Nevanlinna Prize for major contributions to the mathematical aspects of computer science. Dr. Madhu Sudan, an Indian-born computer scientist working at the Massachusetts Institute of Technology (MIT), USA was the recipient of this prestigious prize at the Beijing conference of IMC (2002).

Dr. Madhu Sudan, born at Chennai, got his bachelor's degree in computer science from IIT, Delhi. He received the Nevanlinna Prize for his contributions made in the field of error correcting codes and probabilistically checkable proofs—a way to recast mathematical proofs in computer language for additional checks on its validity—and in non-approximability of optimisation problems.

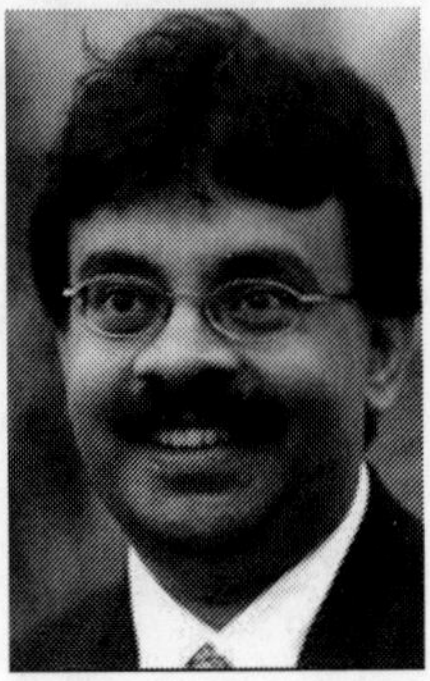

Conclusion

Receiving the Fields Medal award in mathematics is equivalent to the Nobel Prize. No Indian mathematician has received this award so far. The history of the awards is included in articles [1], [2] and [3]. The book mentioned in reference [4] provides more information on the awards while the web sites in the references are also useful. These references are listed lecture-wise at the end of the book.

Lecture 2

Chaos before Cantor

Abstract

In this lecture, we take a cursory review of the logical difficulties which mathematicians have encountered throughout the history of mathematics when they tried to apply methods of finite mathematics to the concept of infinity.

2.1 Introduction

The concept of infinity appears in almost every field of mathematics. Sometimes, its presence is explicit. Sometimes it is not so explicit. Arithmetic and classical algebra deal with numbers. All the numbers taken together form infinite collections. In geometry, we encounter points on a line, lines on a plane, planes in space. These are not only infinite in number, but are also infinite in extent. There is a very important branch of mathematics called mathematical analysis. Its core consists of concepts like limits, continuity, sequences, series, derivation, integration besides many other concepts – all dealing not only with infinitely large quantities but also with infinitely small quantities.

We mortals, however, are equipped to handle only such quantities, whose measure is finite. If we apply our understanding of the finite world to any phenomena having infinitely large or infinitely small extent, we meet chaotic situations.

In this lecture we briefly discuss the problems which ignorance of the proper concept of infinity, create for us.

2.2 Potential Infinity and Actual Infinity

Mathematicians consider two types of infinities—potential infinity and actual infinity. Potential infinity was accepted as a legitimate mathematical object by mathematicians and logicians. But actual infinity was not accepted until German mathematician George Cantor defined the concept. Let us first understand the meaning of potential infinity.

2.2.1 Of what Price is Nothing?

Has anybody heard of a shop where the price of purchasing *nothing* is beyond the capacity of even the richest person in the world!

A British lady wanted to purchase a dog. She visited a shopping mall where dogs of all sizes and breeds were sold.

"How much will I have to pay for this one?", the lady asked the attendant, pointing at a big dog.

"Hundred pounds, Madame", came the reply.

Thinking that it was rather expensive, she turned to a smaller dog and enquired about its price.

"Madame, this one is a bit costly, but I will sell it to you for two hundreds pounds only," he informed.

"Two hundred pounds! for this one! Then how much would I need to pay, if I go for this smaller one?," she asked pointing to a still smaller animal.

"Madame, that one is expensive. It costs 400 pounds."

"My God!" she exclaimed, "The smaller the size I go for, the higher the price you quote. How much will I have to pay, if I leave without purchasing a dog?"

It is a popular belief that women, when compared to men, have better common sense and less mathematical sense. This episode tells us exactly the opposite. The lady in the episode seems to have great mathematical acumen. The answer to her question is infinity! Of course, potential infinity! In schools we try to convince students that $\frac{1}{0}$ is infinity, by showing them that $\frac{1}{0.1} = 10, \frac{1}{0.01} = 100, \ldots, \frac{1}{0.0001} = 10,000, \ldots$ Thus as the denominator diminishes, the quotient grows so that when the denominator becomes zero, the quotient is infinite. This is potential infinity.[1] It is reasonable then to ask, what is the sum of all natural numbers: $1 + 2 + 3 + \ldots = ?$

It is obvious that the sum $1+2+3+4$ is greater than the sum $1+2+3$. More generally, the sum $1 + 2 + \ldots + (n + 1)$ is greater than the sum $1+2+\ldots+n$, whatever the natural number n may be. The sum increases

[1]Strictly speaking, for mathematicians, $\frac{1}{0}$ is undefined. Algebraists, dealing with only finite operations, say that 0 has no "multiplicative inverse". Analysts say that the limit of $\frac{1}{x}$ as x approaches 0 does not existit fluctuates between plus infinity and minus infinity.

with the natural number n. Since there is no greatest natural number, n can increase without bounds and so does the sum of the first n natural numbers, though at any given stage it is finite. Therefore, it is reasonable to assume that the sum of all natural numbers is infinite and that it is a potential infinity. But how many terms are there in the sum of all natural numbers? In other words: what is the totality of all natural numbers? Here also the answer is infinity, but here it is actual infinity. For, here we consider all the natural numbers in one go.

There are several theories of the origin of the universe that we live in. According to one theory, the universe started with a big explosion or a big bang and that it continues to expand in all directions. This is known as the Big Bang Theory. There is another theory called the Steady State Theory. According to this theory, the universe has no beginning. It has no end. If we accept the Big Bang Theory, the life of the universe is infinite. But it is potentially infinite. At any given instant, its age will be finite. On the other hand, if we subscribe to the Steady State Theory, then again the life of the universe is infinite, but it will be actual infinity.

Mathematicians and logicians were able to somehow work with potential infinity. But actual infinity was a hopeless case. At least that was the feeling of a practitioner of mathematics till the late nineteenth century.

A famous mathematician, Euler, started denoting infinity by the symbol ∞, which is now universally used. Renowned astrophysicist, Sir Arthur Eddington cautioned his fellow physicists that ∞ was a love knot with which no physicist should get entangled. Greek philosopher–logician Zeno (300 BCE) was probably the first to notice how actual infinity defies finite logic.

2.3 Zeno's Paradoxes

Zeno makes several ingenious statements. We consider here four of them.

1. Achilles, the mighty and fast, cannot overtake the tortoise, the slowest creature on the earth, if there is race between the two.
2. Two horses cannot run towards each other.
3. It is impossible to cross a field. It takes infinite time to accomplish the task.
4. An arrow in motion is actually at rest.

Let us try to understand his arguments.

2.3.1 Achilles and the Tortoise

Suppose there is a race between Achilles and a tortoise. Achilles, the hero of *Iliad*, being several times faster than the tortoise, offers a small concession to the poor creature. Just as a tennis champion, who usually plays with the right hand, may play with the left in a game against a novice, Achilles stands a few steps behind the tortoise, when the race starts. Zeno claims then, that, Achilles cannot win the race.

Suppose Achilles is at the point A and the tortoise is at the point T, when the race starts. If Achilles is to overtake the tortoise, then he first has to reach the tortoise. For this to happen, both Achilles and the tortoise will have to be at the same point say P, at the same time. In other words, in the same length of time, Achilles will have to cover the length AP, while the tortoise will have to cover the length TP.

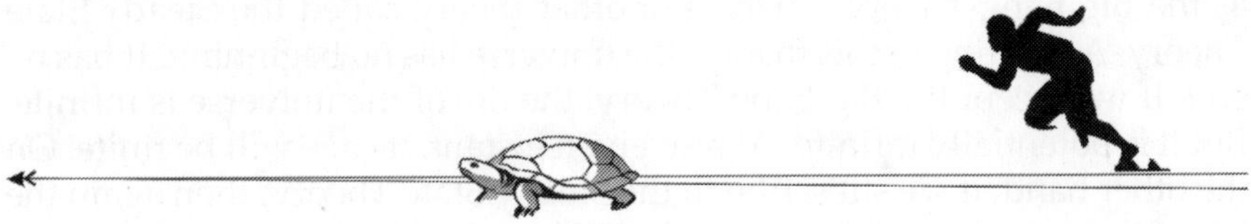

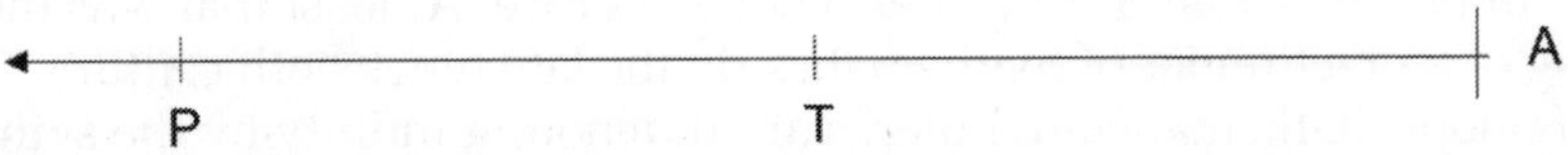

Since the line segment TP is a part of the line segment AP, and since the whole is always greater than its part, the segment AP has more points in it than the segment TP.[2] Thus Achilles can win the race, only if he crosses more points than the tortoise in the above time interval. Is it possible? Zeno's answer is an emphatic "no". Let us see, why.

Zeno's argument is based on the following "self-evident" facts.

i. An instant is the last indestructible part of time. There is no fractional instant.

ii. A point is the last indestructible part of a line. There is no fraction of a point.

If Achilles is faster than the tortoise, he has to cover more points per instant than the tortoise does. Does he cover (say) two points while the tortoise covers just one, in an instant? If the answer is positive, then the next question arises. How much time does he take to cross a point? Half an instant? Since a half-instant does not exist, Achilles must cover only a point in an instant. Similarly, the assumption that the tortoise, being slow, may be taking two instants to cross a point is absurd. Thus, both

[2]Euclid's famous book *Elements* is based on ten self-evident truths. One of them states that the "whole is greater than its part". The importance given to *Elements* in 18th century Europe could be rivalled only by *The Bible*.

Achilles and the tortoise cover just a point per instant. Clearly, Achilles cannot win over the tortoise, as he is required to cover "more points" in the same "amount" of instants.

2.3.2 Horses cannot Meet

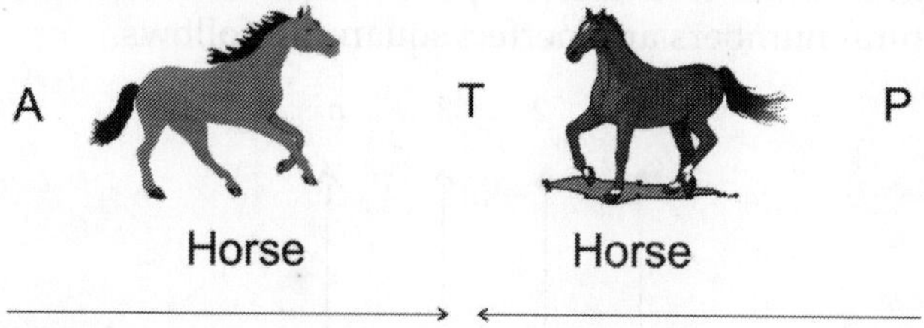

If two horses approach each other, crossing a point per instant, then effectively, they are crossing two points per instant. As explained above, this is impossible. Hence, the two horses running towards each other cannot meet.

2.3.3 You cannot Cross a Field

In order to cross a field you will have to cross half of it. But in order to cross the half, you will have to cross half of the half, i.e., 1/4 of the distance. Repeating the argument, you will have to cover infinitely many distances $1/2$, $1/4$, $1/8$, $\ldots 1/2^n$, ….

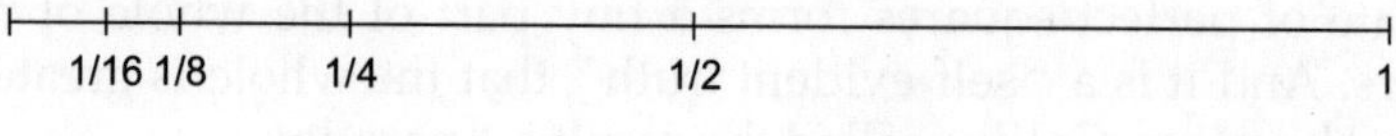

To cover any positive distance, you will need some positive time duration, however small. Hence to cover infinitely many distances you will need infinite time. Clearly, this is not possible for a mortal.

2.3.4 Arrow in Motion is at Rest

Suppose an arrow leaves a bow and hits the target at 300 metres in 10 seconds. If we assume that the velocity is uniform, it is obvious that it will be at the distance of 150 metres at the end of 5 seconds. More generally, given an instant of time, we will be able to state precisely the point at which the arrow will be found. (This is possible even if the velocity under consideration is not uniform). Clearly, if we are able to locate the point precisely at each instant of time, the arrow must be static at that point at that instant. Thus, an arrow in flight is actually at rest.

2.4 Galileo's Paradox

One of the great astrophysicists, Galileo (1564–1642), attempted to count integers which were perfect squares. He observed that every square integer corresponds to a unique natural number and every natural number corresponds to a unique perfect square. Thus he could form pairs of natural numbers and perfect squares as follows.

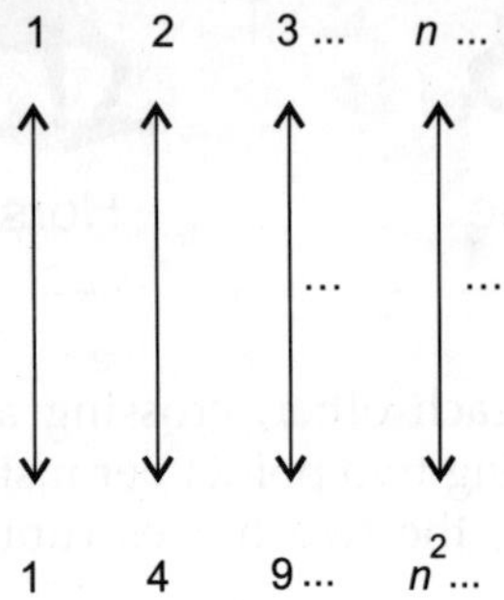

If in a hall there are hundred chairs, and all the chairs are occupied and there is nobody in the hall without a chair, then it is obvious that there are hundred persons in the hall. We arrive at this conclusion without physically counting the persons. For, we know, from the property of pairs, that there are as many persons as there are chairs. This logic compelled Galilio to conclude that there are as many perfect squares as there are natural numbers. But Galileo was not happy with this conclusion. The aggregate of perfect squares forms a tiny part of the whole of natural numbers. And it is a " self-evident truth " that the whole is greater than its part. Therefore, Galileo called the result a " paradox ".

2.5 Tristram Shandy's Plight

Tristram Shandy is a hero of a novel of the same name by the 18th century novelist, Laurence Sterne. Shandy intends to write an autobiography. But he encounters a peculiar problem. His life is too eventful to complete the work. It takes him one year to cover the events of a day. Obviously, however hard he may try, he cannot finish the task.

Suppose Maruti (Hanuman) begins to write his autobiography. His life is also very eventful. He had to fight Indra, the king of gods, for he tried to swallow the sun as soon as he was born. He fought many wars, including the great war between Ram and Ravana. He witnessed the great war on Kurukshetra. Thus, Maruti may also need one year to describe the events that occured in the span of a day. But Maruti is immortal. He may complete the first day's account during the first year of his life. Second day's in the second year, . . ., nth day's in the nth year.

Does this mean that there are as many days as there are years in the life of Maruti?

Bertrand Russell (1872–1970) called this the Tristram Shandy's Paradox.

2.6 World out of Nothing

Italian mathematician Guido Grandi (1671–1742) in his book *Quadratura Circuli et Hyperbolae* (1703), discussed the result of adding 1 and −1 alternately taken infinitely many times:

$$1 + (-1) + 1 + (-1) + \ldots.$$

If we apply the rules of arithmetic, while calculating the sum, then we arrive at very strange results. Let us denote the sum as S. Then

$$S = 1 + (-1) + 1 + (-1) + \ldots.$$

Associating 1 and −1 in pairs and using the property of 0, we easily get

$$S = (1 + (-1)) + (1 + (-1)) + \ldots = 0 + 0 + \ldots = 0.$$

Thus it seems reasonable to assume that the sum is 0. However if we associate the terms a little differently, we have

$$S = 1 + ((-1) + 1) + ((-1) + 1) + \ldots = 1 + 0 + 0 + \ldots = 1.$$

If we use the following combination of associativity, commutativity and 0, we have

$$\begin{aligned}S &= 1 + \{[(-1) + 1] + [(-1) + 1] + \ldots\}\\ &= 1 + \{[1 + (-1)] + [(1 + (-1)] + \ldots\}\\ &= 1 + \{1 + [(-1) + 1] + [(-1) + 1] + \ldots\}\\ &= 1 + \{1 + 0 + \ldots\} = 2.\end{aligned}$$

Using similar arguments repeatedly, we can prove S to be equal to any natural number. Let us now write

$$\begin{aligned}S &= (1 + (-1)) + (1 + (-1)) + \ldots\\ &= ((-1) + 1) + ((-1) + 1) + \ldots\\ &= (-1) + \{(1 + (-1)) + (1 + (-1)) + \ldots\}\end{aligned}$$

$$= -1 + \{0 + 0 + \ldots\}$$

$$= 1.$$

Thus, using different combinations of the rules applied above, we can show that S is equal to any integer—positive, negative or zero. But the story does not end here.

Consider the following binomial theorem:

$$(1+x)^n = 1 + nx + \left[\frac{n(n-1)}{2}\right] x^2 + \ldots\ldots + nx^{n-1} + x^n. \qquad (1)$$

If we set $n = -1$, then the above expression yields the following infinite sum called a series:

$$\frac{1}{1+x} = (1+x)^{-1} = 1 - x + x^2 - x^3 + \ldots \qquad (2)$$

Putting $x = 1$, we get

$$\frac{1}{2} = 1 - 1 + 1 - 1 + \ldots$$

Therefore $S = \frac{1}{2}$.

If we multiply both sides by -1, then we get

$$-\frac{1}{2} = -1 + 1 - 1 + 1 \ldots$$

$$= ((-1) + 1) + ((-1) + 1) + \ldots$$

$$= (1 + (-1)) + (+1 + (-1)) + \ldots$$

$$= (1 + (-1) + 1 + (-1) + \ldots$$

$$= S.$$

Therefore, Grandi feels that any rational number could be derived from S. The "original" and "obvious" value of S is 0. Therefore Grandi claims that the world is created out of nothing.[3]

This claim has been supported by the famous mathematician Gottfried Wilhelm Leibniz (1646–1716). In fact, he further added that Grandi's conclusion may sound metaphysical, but there is more metaphysical truth in mathematics than is generally believed.

[3]Interestingly, Gottlob Frege (1848–1925) constructed natural numbers starting from the empty set and arrived at the same conclusion. However this contradicts the Indian ethos that "something" cannot be born out of "nothing".

2.7 Negative is Greater than Infinity

One of the most prolific mathematician, Leonard Euler (1707–1783), when confronted with infinity arrived at equally strange conclusions.

Consider equation (1) when $n = -2$; we obtain the following infinite series.

$$\frac{1}{(1+x)^2} = (1+x)^{-2} = 1 - 2x + 3x^2 - 4x^3 + \ldots.$$

Substituting $x = -1$ yields

$$\frac{1}{0} = 1 + 2 + 3 + 4 + \ldots.$$

This is an acceptable proposition, if we assume $(1/0)$ is infinity. Euler invented the symbol ∞ for infinity,

Thus $\infty = 1 + 2 + 3 + \ldots.$

Replacing $-x$ for x in (2) we get

$$\frac{1}{1-x} = 1 + x + x^2 + x^3 + \ldots.$$

Consider this series when $x = 2$. Then we have

$$-1 = 1 + 2 + 4 + 8 + \ldots.$$

Therefore Euler argues that

$$-1 = 1 + 2 + 4 + 8 + \ldots > 1 + 2 + 3 + 4 + \ldots$$

$$= \infty.$$

Thus the infinite sum $1 + 2 + 4 + 8 + \ldots\ldots$ which is a part of the sum $1 + 2 + 3 + 4 + \ldots\ldots$ is greater than the whole, and negative numbers are greater than infinity.

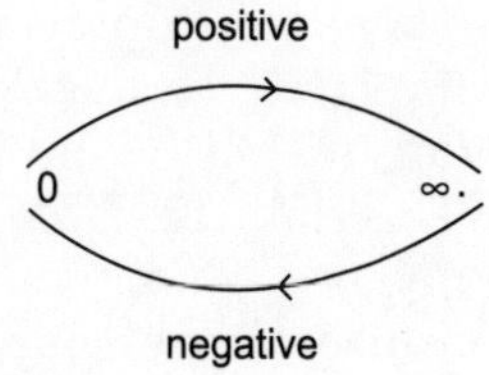

It is strange but true that western mathematicians of the eighteenth century were not at ease with negative numbers. This may be attributed to the legacy obtained from the Greeks, who learnt numbers through geometry. Some of Euler's contemporary mathematicians were of the view that there are two types of negative numbers— negative numbers having values less than 0 and those having values greater than infinity. If we have to arrange the numbers linearly, then we needed to have the two types. Euler suggested a circular arrangement of real numbers, where both 0 and ∞ separate the negative from the positive numbers, so that the same negative number would be less than 0 and greater than ∞ simultaneously, as indicated in the figure.

This had an additional advantage: 0 being both positive and negative, it would be less as well as greater than ∞. Euler was also of the view that $2/0$ is twice as big as $1/0$. Considering the parodoxes ranging from Zeno's statements to Euler's views, we can see that there had been total confusion abut the nature of infinity till the last quarter of the nineteenth century.

Conclusion

The ignorance about the nature of infinity was so universal, that, in the words of mathematician Morris Kline (1908–1992), "Newton, Liebnitz, Bernoulli, Euler, d'Alembert, Lagrange, and several 18th century men struggled with infinite series. They perpetrated all sorts of blunders, made false proofs and drew incorrect conclusions; they even gave arguments that, now with hind sight, we are obliged to call ludicrous."

The reference given in the end of the book provide interesting information on this topic.

Lecture 3

Order Out of Chaos

Abstract

In this lecture we explain, with several illustrations, how the concept of set and the principle of one-to-one correspondence provide new and clear insight into the nature of infinity and resolve the long-standing paradoxes discussed in Lecture 2.

We also obtain, in an informal manner, the cardinalities of sets which frequently occur in mathematics.

3.1 Introduction

We have seen in Lecture 2 how chaotic the situation was in different areas of mathematics when confronted with the concept of infinity. In the last quarter of the nineteenth century, German mathematician George Cantor was successful in creating order out of the chaos. What Cantor achieved was nothing short of a revolution in mathematics. Its impact on mathematics can only be compared with that of the invention of zero and the decimal system. Once Cantor created the beautiful theory of sets, mathematics never looked the same. It gave the subject a very sound footing. Never before had it looked so rigorous, so precise, so aesthetically appealing as it did, after the advent of the concept of sets. At the same time, the theory gave mathematics such a tremendous boost, that the amount of mathematics created in the last one hundred years is much more than that created in all the previous years known to humanity. The concept of sets liberated mathematics from the narrow field of numbers, thus increasing its applicability severalfold. Mathematics is now being used more extensively in almost all branches of human knowledge.

Our objective in this lecture, however, is very modest: To understand how Cantor tackled the problem of infinity that was evading a perfect solution for thousands of years.

Let us recollect, what we mean by the word " infinity ".

3.2 How Big is Infinity?

A two-and-half-year old boy knows how to count up to two. If we give him one candy, he will recognise that he has one. If we give him two candies and ask, "How many candies do you have?", "Two" is the normal answer. But if we give him three candies or more, and ask the same question, then " many " will probably be the answer. For he cannot count beyond two.

In the eighteenth century, Europeans exploring Southwest Africa encountered a tribe they called, the Hottentots. It was believed that nobody in the tribe could count beyond three. Therefore, anything beyond three was " many " for a Hottentot. Clearly, the numbers two or three are not big numbers.

But we know big numbers since antiquity. The story of Sissa Ben Dahir is well known. The king Shirhan was very pleased with Dahir, who had invented the game of chess. He wanted to give a befitting reward to Dahir. Mathematical wizard as he must have been, Dahir requested the king to place one grain of wheat in the first square of a chess board, two in the second square, four in the third and in this way go on doubling the number of grains, till all the sixty-four squares are filled, and give that much wheat to him as a gift. If we assume that there are 5,000,000 grains in a bushel and that the yearly wheat production in the world is 2,000,000,000 bushels, then it would take 2000 years to meet Dahir's demand. Thus, Dahir basically asked for monopoly rights to collect all the wheat in the world for two thousand years! But this is a small number compared to the number of protons in the universe. Sir Arthur Eddington has calculated the number of protons in the universe to be the following 80-digit number.

15, 747, 724, 136, 275, 002, 577, 605, 653, 961, 181, 555, 468, 044, 717, 914, 527, 116, 709, 336, 231, 425, 076, 185, 631, 031, 276.

The number is really big. If we start counting from 1 to reach this number and keep on counting day and night, generation after generation, we will not be able to complete even 15% of the work before life on earth comes to an end.

But we know still bigger numbers. For example the largest known prime number is $2^{756839} - 1$! If it is written in the normal form, it will take more than seven pages of a newspaper. But this number, though very big, is as far away from infinity as it is from the number 1.

Consider the following dialogue between two fighting boys. Before they come to actual blows, there is a battle of words. "I will give you a big punch", says one boy. "I am not sitting idle. I will give you two punches", says the other. "Then I will give three punches"….. These threats continue for some time till one, who is probably more intelligent than the other, declares. "I will give you one punch more than the number of punches I receive from you". The other boy also repeats the same threat. This is probably the first encounter with infinity in the life of children. They realise here, that the numbers do not end – one can always threaten to give more punches than the other boy. For any number n, there is a greater number $n+1$.

According to Indian mythology, Lord Krishna once gave a magical kaleidoscope to Yudhishthir to divert his attention from his brothers. When Yudhishthir looked into the kaleidoscope, he found another Yudhishthir inside, who was looking through a kaleidoscope in which he found another Yudhishthir looking through a kaleidoscope. The original Yudhishthir started counting his replicas and lost himself in counting. Even the fastest computer in the world cannot count the number of replicas of Yudhishthir in the magical kaleidoscope.

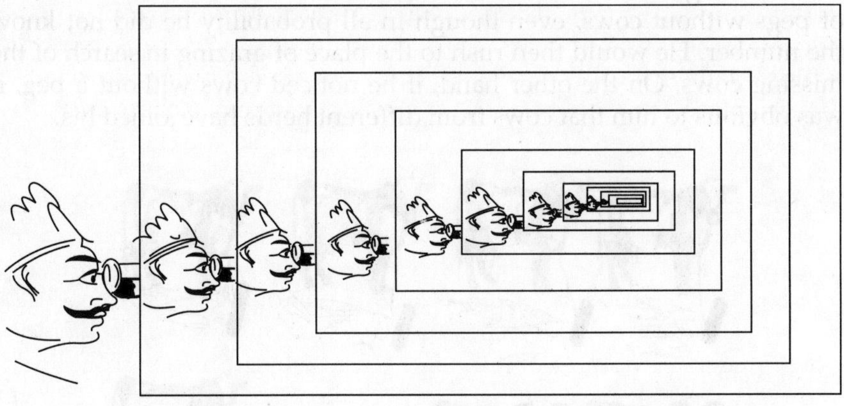

Number of replicas of Yudhishthir in the magical kaleidoscope

All of us must have seen a talcum powder container on which a beautiful girl is painted holding a container of the same brand of talcum powder on which is painted a girl holding a container. Even the most gifted artist in the world cannot complete the picture on the talcum powder container. For the number of replicas and the number of pictures are infinite. They grow while counting is still in process. Infinity is not a number which is difficult to count. It is something which is impossible to count. The difficulty does not lie in the individual's ability, it lies in the very nature of the concept.

3.3 Keeping Account Without Counting

Human intelligence lies in the capacity of finding the difference in seemingly identical situations and commonality in seemingly different situations. Many times, the latter is more difficult to notice than the former. Cantor's genius lay in finding a commonality between his problem and that of the primitive caveman. He observed that although the primitive caveman might have not known how to count beyond three, he did know how to deal with numbers beyond three.

He might be taking, say hundred cows in the morning for grazing and returning with them in the evening. He may not have known the total number of cows in his herd but he definitely managed to bring back his whole herd.

How did he ensure that precisely hundred cows had returned—not more, not less? He used a simple trick. He fixed hundred pegs on the ground and tied precisely one cow to each peg. In the morning, he untied the cows and took them to the grazing place. In the evening, he performed the same exercise in the reverse order—tying one cow to each peg. If some pegs remained without cows, he concluded that some cows were missing. The number of missing cows was the same as the number of pegs without cows, even though in all probability he did not know the number. He would then rush to the place of grazing in search of the missing cows. On the other hand, if he noticed cows without a peg, it was obvious to him that cows from different herds have joined his.

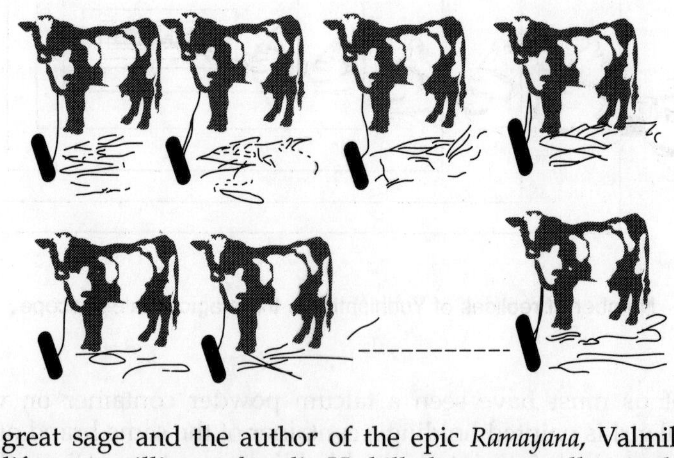

The great sage and the author of the epic *Ramayana*, Valmiki in his former life was an illiterate bandit. He killed stray travellers in the jungle and robbed them. He did not know counting but he did keep an account of those whom he had killed. He placed one pebble in a jar for each of his victim. The primitive caveman formed pairs of a cow and a peg. Valmiki formed pairs of a victim and a pebble. In technical language, this method is called a one-to-one correspondence. Pairing is a procedure which establishes a one-to-one correspondence between two different collections. Cantor thought that since he was in no better position than a primitive caveman when faced with infinity, he should use the principle of one-to-one correspondence to understand infinite collections. This created order out of chaos. All great ideas are simple and this one is no exception. This simple idea opened, in the words of David Hilbert, the gates of paradise for mathematicians.

The application of one-to-one correspondence reveals many secrets of an infinite collection.

3.4 Magic Auditorium

Suppose in an auditorium of capacity, say, 500 persons, we invite 500 persons. Let us assume that all of them have accepted the invitation. At the eleventh hour we realise that we have forgotten a very very important person. It is necessary to "some how" accommodate him. But at the same time it will not be proper for us to deny entry to a bonafide guest-pass-holder. This problem has no graceful solution in the present situation.

But suppose we have an auditorium with infinitely many chairs and tickets for all the chairs are sold, when the problem of the VVIP is noticed. This problem can be solved by a small announcement as follows:

"Please read the seat number n as $n+1$. The inconvenience caused by the printing error is deeply regretted."

The holder of seat number 1, then, will move to seat number 2, that of seat number 2, will move to the seat number 3 .... And thus everybody will get a seat and we still have seat number 1 vacant. It can be offered to the VVIP.

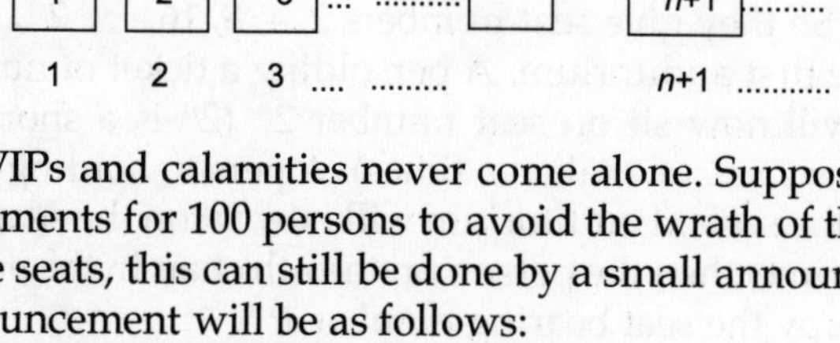

Usually VVIPs and calamities never come alone. Suppose we need to make arrangements for 100 persons to avoid the wrath of the VIP. In the hall of infinite seats, this can still be done by a small announcement. This time the announcement will be as follows:

"Please read the seat number n as $n + 100$..."

Then the occupant of seat number 1 will occupy seat number 101, that of seat number 2, will occupy seat number 102,. . .. Thus the first 100 seats will be available to the VIP and his cronies. Obviously the number 100 can be replaced by any natural number n.

When the news spreads that in the auditorium, seats are available even at the last minute, everybody will try to enter at the last minute. Suppose all the seats are booked and an equal number is standing outside in a queue. We need not worry. We simply make the following announcement:

"Please read seat number n as $2n$."

Then the owner of seat number 1 will go to seat number 2, that of 2 will occupy seat number 4, that of 3, will take seat number 6..., everybody will get a seat, and we still have infinitely many seats vacant, where numbers are odd, i.e. 1, 3, 5, 7.... They can be given to the persons in the queue.

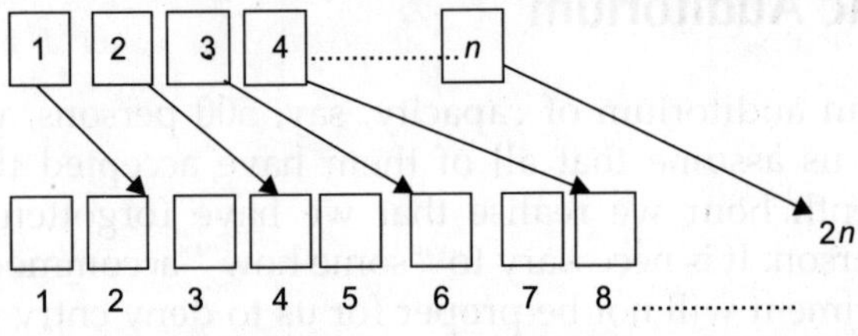

Now suppose this wonderful property of an infinite auditorium tempts an unscrupulous businessman to build an infinite chain of auditoriums, without proper sanctions from the municipal corporation. And one fine morning, an upright and uncompromising officer is appointed by the corporation (such accidents do take place occasionally). The officer orders the demolition of all unauthorised buildings. Clearly all the infinite auditoriums, except the original one, are demolished. The owner of the auditoriums is in a fix. He has already arranged a premium show of a big budget movie, in all the auditoriums simultaneously. All the tickets are sold. If he does not honour his commitment, he will lose not only money but also his name. Moreover there may be a big pandemonium and hence cause a law and order problem. So a team of experts is appointed to solve the problem of accommodation. And they come up with a beautiful solution – probably some of the experts are good at mathematics. They know that the collection of prime numbers (that is a natural number greater than 1 and divisible only by itself and 1) 2, 3, 5, 7, 11, 13, 17, . . .is without end. So they give seat numbers 2, 4, 8, 16, . . ., 2^n, . . .to the ticket holders of the first auditorium. A persolding a ticket of number n in that auditorium will now sit on seat number 2^n (2^n is a short form for the number $2 \times 2 \times 2 \times \ldots \times 2$ taken n times). A person holding a ticket of seat number n in the second auditorium will now sit on the seat number 3^n. If p is the mth prime, then the person on the nth chair in the mth auditorium will now occupy the seat bearing number P^n.

In this arrangement, no two persons will get the same seat number. This is so because of the following property of primes. If p and q are two primes and n and m are two natural numbers, then $p^n = q^m$ will simply mean $p = q$ and $n = m$. Clearly $p = q$ ensures that the auditoriums are the same, and $n = m$ means that the seat numbers are the same.

Moreover, infinitely many seats will still be vacant. For example, seat 1 is obviously vacant. But any seat whose number can be divided by more than one distinct prime (for example 6, which can be divided by two primes 2 and 3, 90 which can be divided by three primes 2, 3, 5 etc.) are vacant. Of course there are still more elegant and easily computable ways. For example, an occupant of nth seat in the mth auditorium may be given $2^n\ 3^m$th seat. Since $2^n\ 3^m = 2^r 3^s$ holds only when $n = r$ and $m = s$, no two persons will get the same seat in this scheme also. Replacing 2 and 3 by any other two prime numbers p and q $(p \neq q)$, we get a different scheme of allotment.

Infinity has many such unbelievable properties. For example, suppose the management decides to present a small watch to everybody attending the premier show and contracts for the supply of these watches. Obviously the contractor would like to maximise his profit. So he brings watches only for half of the audience and still presents a watch to everybody, and then he repents. He could have done the job with much less! By this time, we know how this can be done.

The device of one-to-one correspondence tells us how to arrive at the precise definition of infinity.

3.5 Precise Definition of Infinity

If we consider a one-to-one correspondence between two collections of objects, then obviously we need to have two collections and a rule to pair off the objects in the collections. In the language of mathematics, these collections are called sets. Thus a set, according to Cantor, is a collection or an aggregate of any definite and distinguishable things which a human mind can think of. It is a collection of objects under study. These objects may be concrete things like chairs or abstract ideas like numbers. The objects are called elements or members of the set. A set is usually denoted by capital letters like A, B, or X, Y. Elements of a set are denoted by small letters a, b, x, y,... A mathematician's way of writing the sentence "a is an element of the set A" is "$a \in A$". It is read as "a is in A" or "a belong to A". If a set A consists of elements $a_1, a_2 \ldots, a_n$ then we write $A = \{a_1, a_2, \ldots a_n\}$ or alternatively $A = \{a_i | i = 1, 2, 3 \ldots, n\}$. The set C of all chairs may be written as

$$C = \{x | x \text{ is a chair}\}.$$

More generally, if X is a set of elements x, satisfying a property P, then we write $X = \{x|P(x)\}$. However to keep things simple, we will avoid using these symbols as far as possible.

The principle of one-to-one correspondence is applicable not only to infinite sets but to any set. When we say we have five apples, we mean that the set of apples is in one-to-one correspondence with the set of fingers of one (normal) hand. In fact, by the number 5 we mean the property which is common to all sets which are in one-to-one correspondence with the set of fingers of one hand. Likewise, by hundred we mean that property which is common to all sets which are in one-to-one correspondence with the set of symbols $1, 2, 3, \ldots, 99, 100$. Cantor names this common property as the cardinality or cardinal number of a set. Accordingly, two sets will have the same cardinality if and only if we can establish a one-to-one correspondence between the elements of the two sets.

This way one can attach cardinality to every set. We start with a set which has no element. This set is like an empty box. So it is called an empty set. An empty set is denoted by a symbol Φ. Since Φ has no element, we define 0 (zero) to be the cardinality of Φ. The cardinality of a set whose sole element is Φ, is denoted by $\{\Phi\}$. The cardinality of the set $\{\Phi\}$ is called 1. The number 2 is the cardinality of the set $\{\Phi, \{\Phi\}\}$ – the set whose only elements are Φ and $\{\Phi\}$. This way all natural numbers can be defined step by step. The cardinality of the set of all natural numbers is denoted by the first Hebrew letter $\aleph$ with subscript 0. Thus $\aleph_0$ (aleph naught) is the cardinality of the set of natural numbers. Since natural numbers are used for counting, the cardinality of any set whose cardinality is either a natural number or $\aleph_0$, is called a countable set.

It can be seen from several examples that the set of natural numbers (which we denote by the letter N) is infinite. But we are not given any rigorous definition of infinity. What separates N from finite sets like $\{1, 2, 3, \ldots n\}$? Human intelligence lies in noticing a common property in seemingly different objects and differences in seemingly identical objects. It is proof of Cantor's genius that he noticed the commonality and the difference between finite and infinite sets. Cantor attaches cardinality to every set, be it finite or infinite. To understand the difference between finity and infinity however, we need the concept of a subset.

From every set we can obtain a new set by deleting some elements. This new set is called a subset of the given set. Thus if $A = \{1, 2, 3, \ldots, 100\}$, then the set $B = \{2, 3, \ldots, 100\}$ is its subset. For B is obtained by deleting 1 from A. The set of even integers $C = \{2, 4, 6, \ldots, 98, 100\}$ is also a subset of A. For C is obtained by deleting odd integers from A. The set Φ is a subset of every set. For it is obtained by deleting all elements of that set. The word " some " also includes 0 (zero). Hence every set is a subset of itself, for it is obtained by deleting zero number of elements. Thus if X is a set then, Φ and X are always subsets of X. But they are called improper subsets of X. All others are called proper subsets of X.

Cantor noticed that if X is finite, then the cardinality of every proper subset of X is less than the cardinality of X. For example, the cardinality of A described above is 100, that of B is 99, and that of C is 50. The cardinality of every proper subset of A is less than 100. But this does not happen with infinite sets. As seen in the example of the magic auditorium, the cardinality of N and the subset S obtained from N by deleting 1 is the same. The cardinality of the subset $T = \{2, 4, 6, 8, 10, \ldots\}$ of even positive integers is also the same as that of N. Of course some subsets may have different cardinality. For example, the cardinality of $\{1\}$, which is definitely a subset of N is different from that of N. But N does have a proper subset of the same cardinality as its own. This never happens with finite sets. Cantor, therefore, gives the following definition of an infinite set.

DEFINITION: An infinite set is a set which has a proper subset of the same cardinality as its own.

Euclid has given five axioms or self-evident truths in his book on geometry. The fifth axiom is: The whole is greater than its parts. The set of even integers is obviously a part of N. But it is as big as the whole N. So a finite set is a set where Euclid's fifth axiom holds, and an infinite set is a set where Euclid's fifth axiom fails to hold.

3.6 Resolution of Paradoxes

Cantor's definition of an infinite set and his method of one-to-one correspondence resolve several paradoxes stated in Lecture 2.

3.6.1 Galileo's Paradox

Galileo observed (See Lecture 2, Section 2.4) that the set of perfect squares {1, 4, 9, 25, ...} is in one-to-one correspondence with the set of natural numbers. There is no paradox in his observation. In fact, he had proved that the set of natural numbers is infinite. His unflinching faith in the Euclidean axiom led him to think that it was a paradox.

3.6.2 Tristram Shandy's Paradox

This also is no paradox (See Lecture 2, Section 2.5). In an infinite time frame, the set of number of years and that of the days have the same cardinality.

3.6.3 Achilles' Paradox

Here the claim (See Lecture 2, Section 2.3.1) for the paradox rests on three assumptions.

a. An instant is the smallest indestructible part of time.

b. A point is the smallest indestructible part of a line.

c. A bigger line has more points than a smaller line.

Since the assumptions (a) and (b) are essentially definitions of the words "instant" and "point", we turn to the assumption (c).

The assumption (c) is based on Euclid's fifth axiom. Since a line segment however short it may be, contains infinitely many points, Euclid's axiom cannot be applied to the "number" of points in a line segment. Therefore, whether two line segments have equal or different "number" of points on them will have to be tested by the method of one-to-one correspondence. The fact that one line segment is shorter than the other, does not prove that any other correspondence between points is not one-to-one.

Let AB and CD be two line segments, AB being shorter than CD. Join C to A and D to B. By extending the lines CA and DB, let us complete the triangle COD. Let a line through O cut the line AB at P and CD at Q internally. As the line "sweeps" the triangle, starting from the "initial position" OAC, to the final position OBD, P varies from A to B and Q varies from C to D, giving us the required one-to-one correspondence between the points of the two line segments. Hence the number (cardinality) of points on both lines is the same. Thus the assumption (c) is not true. Since Achilles does not cross more points in order to overtake the tortoise, there is no paradox.

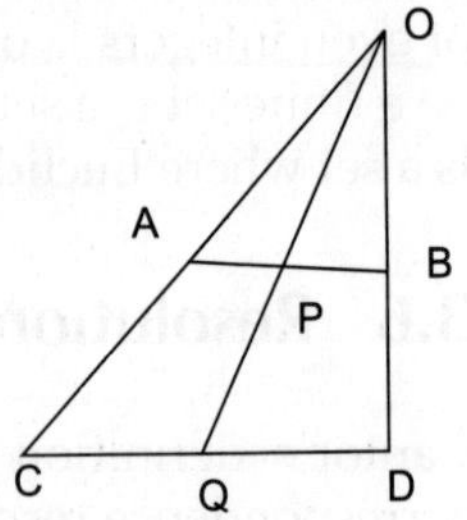

3.6.4 Static Arrow's Paradox

Cantor's set theory puts a physical phenomena in more precise mathematical terms. Zeno's paradox of the arrow (See Lecture 2, Section 2.3.4) says that there is a one-to-one correspondence between "time-points" (instants) and "space-points" (position of the arrow). But the fact that the arrow is exactly at one point at any given instant of time does not mean that the arrow does not move. Zeno's error, in the words of Bertrand Russell, lies "in inferring (if he did infer) that, because there is no such thing as a state of change, the world is in the same state at any one time as at any other".

3.6.5 Other Paradoxes

The other paradoxes of Zeno are also resolved once Cantor, Dedikind and Weierstrass introduced and perfected the concepts of limits, continuity, convergence, derivatives and integration and through them paved the way to mathematisation of physics on sounder footings. However, this topic is too technical to be discussed here.

3.7 Cardinality of some Well-known Sets

Before acquiring more information about cardinality, it is useful to find the cardinality of sets which occur frequently in any mathematical discussion.

In order to understand the logic of the methods adopted by Cantor to establish one-to-one correspondence between different sets, it is necessary to notice one more aspect of infinity. Cantor observed that the process of counting is actually the process of ordering the objects under consideration. In other words, it is impossible to count unless we put the objects in a specific order. Consider counting a set containing 100 elements. We pick some element and call it the first element and then we pick up another element and call it the second element... and this process of picking is exhausted at the 100th step. It was the genius of Cantor to notice that infinite sets differ from finite sets in one respect other than the violation of Euclid's fifth axiom. If a set has finitely many elements, then the order in which we count them is not important. Any order yields the same number. But this does not happen, when we "count" infinity. Here ordering does matter. If X and Y are two infinite sets then, pairing elements of X and Y in a particular ordering for X and Y may exhibit one-to-one correspondence between the elements of X and those of Y; while in some other ordering, X may be in one-to-one correspondence with a proper subset of Y and not the whole of Y. Therefore, before arriving at the final conclusion of whether two sets have the same cardinality or not, we must pay sufficient attention to the ordering of the sets under consideration. The following examples illustrate this fact.

3.7.1 The Cardinality of Z

The set of all integers is denoted by the symbol Z. Thus

$$Z = \{\ldots, -3, -2, -1, 0, 1, 2, 3, \ldots\}.$$

The set of natural numbers is denoted by N. Thus

$$N = 1, 2, 3, \ldots.$$

Under the usual ordering of integers it is obvious that N is not in one-to-one correspondence with Z. Intuitively it is obvious that Z is twice as big as N. But Cantor's method of one-to-one correspondence shows that intuition is no guarantee of truth. Let us order the elements of Z as indicated by the arrows in the figure.

This is not a usual ordering. Normally, Z has no smallest element or the first element. But here 0 is the first, -1 the second, 1 the third... and thus we establish a one-to-one correspondence between the elements of Z and those of N. Hence the cardinality of Z is $\aleph_0$. There is a less direct way to arrive at the same conclusion. Let S be the set of negative integers. $S = \{-1, -2, -3, \ldots\}$. Clearly the cardinality of N and S is the same. From the example of the auditorium of infinite seats it is clear that by "adding" two countable sets we get a countable set. Therefore "addition" of the set of positive and negative integers together yields a countable set. To this countable set, we just have to add one more element, namely 0, to get Z.

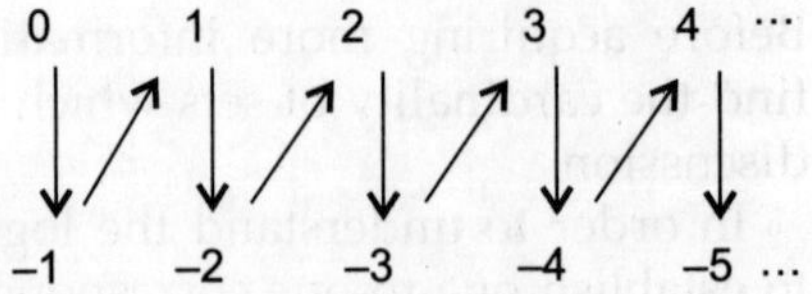

3.7.2 The Cardinality of Pairs of Integers

Consider the set of pairs (m, n), where m and n are natural numbers. It is denoted by the symbol $N \times N$ and consists of the following arrangement of infinite rows and columns.

(1,1)	(1,2)	(1,3)	…
(2,1)	(2,2)	(2,3)	…
(3,1)	(3,2)	(3,3)	…
…	…	…	…

This is obviously a "doubly" infinite sequence of rows and columns Therefore one may be tempted to conclude that the infinity of this set is bigger than the infinity of the set of natural numbers. But, if we arrange the elements in the order indicated by the arrows in the following figure, then we easily notice that they are in one-to-one correspondence with the set of natural numbers.

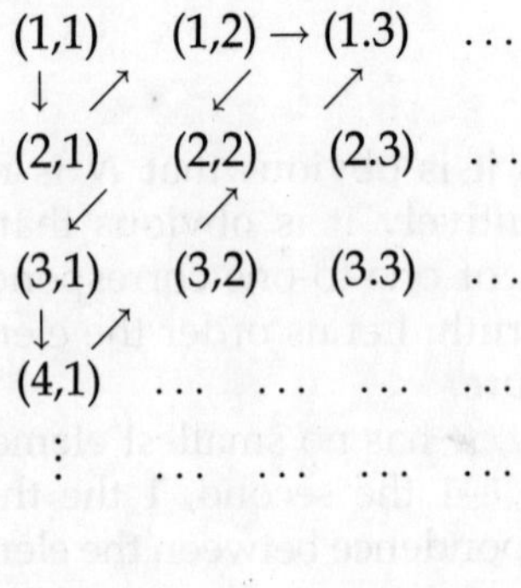

The arrows in the above diagram put the pairs in the following order: The first element is (1,1). This is the pair (m, n), where $m + n = 2$. Then we collect the pairs (m, n), for which $m + n = 3$, then we turn to pairs for which $m + n = 4, \ldots$, etc. in that order. While ordering pairs with the same sum, we select the nearest pair to be the next in sequence. They are indicated by inclined arrows, either rising or falling. When all arrows with the same sum are ordered, then there will be a jump of 1 in the sum. Here, the next pair is indicated by either a horizontal arrow or a vertical arrow. If the previous arrow is falling, then the next term is vertically down. If the previous arrow is rising, then the next term is horizontally to the right.

This matching of ordered pairs of natural numbers with natural numbers themselves is clear from the above figure.

The set of ordered pairs of natural numbers is denoted by $N \times N$. Thus $N \times N = \{(m, n)\}|m, n \in N\}$ is countable. Clearly N (can be replaced by any other countable set; for we are interested only in the "number" of elements in the set and not in the set itself). Thus, more generally, if S and T are countable sets, then so is

$$S \times T = \{(s, t)|s \in S, t \in T\}.$$

3.7.3 Countability of n-tuples

In the above discussion, let us replace S by $N \times N$ and T by N itself. Since both are countable, so is the set $(N \times N) \times N$. But this set can be easily seen to be the "same" as the set of ordered triples $N \times N \times N = \{(a_1, a_2, a_3)|a_i \in N, i = 1, 2, 3\}$. Thus we have proved that the set of ordered triples is countable. Replacing S by $N \times N \times N$ and T by N and arguing on similar lines, we find that the set of 4-tuples is countable. Extending the argument step by step, we conclude that the set of n-tuples

$$\{(a_1, a_2, \ldots, a_n)|a_i \in N, i = 1, 2, 3 \ldots n)\} \text{ is countable.}$$

Clearly, again N can be replaced by any countable set.

3.7.4 Countable Union of Countable Sets

If A and B are two sets then a new set C can be constructed from the sets A and B. The elements of C are all the elements of both A and B. Thus if x is an element of C, then it is either in A or in B or both. The set C is called the union of A and B. The concept can be easily extended to any set of countably many sets. Now let us recall the "rectangular" arrangement of infinitely extended rows and columns. A typical column $(1, m), (2, m), (3, m) \ldots$, may be considered as a countable set of pairs (n, m), $n = 1, 2, 3, \ldots$. Allowing m to assume values $1, 2, 3, \ldots$ we get the set $N \times N$. For this reason $N \times N$ is a countable union of countable sets. Therefore we conclude that the countable union of countable sets is countable.

It is this result which bestows magic properties to the auditorium of infinitely many seats discussed in Lecture 2.

3.7.5 The Set of all Polynomials is Countable

Polynomials constitute a very important part of mathematics. Expressions like $1+x, 1-5x^2, 3+6x+5x^3-7x^8$ are polynomials with integral coefficients. More generally the expressions $a_0+a_1x+a_2x^2+\ldots+a_{n-1}x^{n-1}+a_nx^n$, where $a_0, a_1, \ldots, a_n$ are integers are called polynomials with integral coefficients. Since we are interested only in integral coefficients, we refer to them as just polynomials. If $a_n \neq 0$, then it is called a polynomial of degree n. In particular every integer $a \neq 0$ may be treated as a polynomial of degree 0.

Clearly then, we say that the set of polynomials of degree 0 is countable.

But this is nothing. Consider the set of all polynomials of degree 1. It is the set $S = \{a_0 + a_1x | a_0, a_1 \in Z, a_1 \neq 0\}$. Since x does not play any significant role in determining S, we may identify S with the set of ordered pairs

$$Z \times Z = \{(a_0, a_1) | a_0, a_1 \in Z, a_1 \neq 0\}.$$

Since $Z \times Z$ is countable, the set of all polynomials of degree 1 is countable.

More generally, the set of polynomials of degree n can be identified with the countable set of $(n+1)$-tuples

$$\{(a_0, a_1 \ldots a_n) | a_1 \in Z, a_n \neq 0\}.$$

Therefore if X_n is the set all polynomials of degree n, then X_n is countable for all $n = 1, 2, 3 \ldots$.

The set of all polynomials is then the union of all X_n. Since the countable union of countable sets is countable, the set of all polynomials is countable.

3.7.6 The Set of all Rationals is Countable

Before calculating the cardinality of the set Q of all rational numbers, we state a very useful theorem which looks very obvious, although its proof is not obvious at all. The theorem is known as the Schroeder–Bernstein Theorem. We can use this theorem to compare the cardinalities of two sets without actually matching the elements.

SCHROEDER-BERNSTEIN THEOREM: Two sets A and B have the same cardinality if A is in one-to-one correspondence with a subset of B and B is in one-to-one correspondence with a subset of A.

The result that $N \times N$ and N have the same cardinality can be very elegantly proved by using the Schroeder–Bernstein Theorem. Clearly N is in one-to-one correspondence with a subset of $N \times N$. The set $N \times \{1\}$

is obviously one such subset of $N \times N$. $S = \{2^m 3^n | m, n \in N\}$ is clearly a subset of N. Following the arguments put forward before (Lecture 3, Section 3.4), it can be proved that the correspondence $(m, n) \leftrightarrow 2^m 3^n$ one-to-one from $N \times N$ onto the subset S of N.

Now let us turn to our problem of rational numbers. We first focus our attention on the set Q^+ of all positive rationals. Clearly Q^+ consists of all numbers of the type m/n, where $m, n, \in N$. Of course infinitely many pairs represent the same rational number. For example: 2/3 is represented by $2m/3m$ for any $m \in N$. Therefore, we assume that Q^+ consists of only those quotients m/n, where m and n have no common factor. Under this assumption each element of Q^+ will be uniquely represented by an ordered pair $(m, n) \in N \times N$. Clearly the matching of pair m/n and (m, n) gives a one-to-one correspondence between Q^+ and a subset of $N \times N$. We already know that there is a one-to-one correspondence between the elements of $N \times N$ and N, because $N \times N$ and N have the same cardinality. Combining the two correspondences, we get a one-to-one correspondence between Q^+ and a subset of N. On the other hand, every integer n is a rational number $n/1$. Hence there is one-to-one correspondence between N and a subset of Q^+ namely N itself. Therefore by the Schroeder–Bernstein Theorem, Q^+ and N have the same cardinality. Since negative rational numbers will also have the same cardinality as Q^+ and Q is obtained by adding positive and negative rational numbers together with 0, we conclude, that Q has the same cardinality as N.

3.7.7 The Set of all Algebraic Numbers is Countable

Consider a polynomial $a_0 + a_1 x + \ldots. + a_n x^n$. Here $a_0, a_1, \ldots, a_n$ are integers. If we replace x by any real number, then the expression gives a real number. For example, if we substitute $x = 1$ in $1 + 3x$ we get 4; if we put $x = -2$, we get -5. If for some value of x we get the value of the expression to be 0, then that value of x is called the root of the polynomial. In the present case $x = -\frac{1}{3}$ is the root of the polynomial $1 + 3x$. A real or complex number which is a root of some polynomial (with integral coefficient) is called algebraic. Every rational number m/n is a root of the polynomial $m - nx$ and hence is algebraic. There are irrational algebraic too. For example $\sqrt{2}$ is a root of the polynomial with integral coefficients. $x^2 - 2$, π, $2^{\sqrt{2}}$, e are some examples of numbers which are not the roots of polynomials with integral coefficients. They are called transcendental numbers. Ordinarily, we encounter them less frequently.

By the fundamental theorem of algebra, each polynomial of degree n will not have more than n distinct roots. Since there are only countably many polynomials with integral coefficients, there will be only countably many algebraic numbers.

3.8 Uncountable Sets

3.8.1 The Cardinality of Unit Interval (0,1)

We have seen that (i) the set of natural numbers, (ii) the set of integers, (iii) the set of rational numbers, (iv) the set of n-tuples of natural numbers/integers/rationals, and (v) the set of algebraic numbers, all have the same cardinality. Since we use the natural numbers for counting, we call the cardinality of these sets as countable cardinality. However when one finds that a countable union of countable sets is countable, one really wonders, if there is any infinite set of cardinality other than which is countable. If there were none, Cantor's theory of cardinal numbers would have been devoid of any real meaning. Fortunately this is not the case. We now know that there are infinitely many distinct infinite cardinal numbers. In the year 1880, Cantor proved that there are infinite sets which are not in one-to-one correspondence with N and hence their cardinality is uncountable. The set of all real numbers greater than 0 and less than 1 is one such set.

Cantor's proof is short and elegant. It is considered as one of the most beautiful proofs in mathematics.

The set of real numbers strictly lying between 0 and 1 is called the open unit interval and is denoted by (0, 1). It is clear that the set $S = \{1/n | n \in N\}$ is a subset of (0,1). The matching $n \leftrightarrow 1/n$ establishes a one-to-one correspondence between N and the subset S of (0,1). Cantor shows that any attempt at ordering the elements of (0,1) as the first element, second element, third element, ...leads to contradiction .

Any infinite decimal expression, say 0.2158...represents a real number between 0 and 1. On the other hand, any number between 0 and 1 can be given a unique infinite decimal representation. The uniqueness is disturbed only in one situation, when there is an infinite chain of zeros. For example, 1/4 has two infinite decimal expressions: 0.25000... and 0.24999.... To ensure uniqueness, we decide to choose an infinite chain of the second type. Irrational numbers have an infinite decimal expression with no regular pattern, for example $\pi/4$ is 0.785398... (The irrational number π has been computed up to few million terms and no regular pattern has been observed and naturally so).

Cantor says that if these numbers form a countable set, then they must be in one-to-one correspondence with N and therefore we must be able to list them as the first number, second number.....etc. Suppose the following is one such list:

$$
\begin{array}{llll}
1.\ 0. & a_{11} & a_{12} & a_{13}\cdots \\
2.\ 0. & a_{21} & a_{22} & a_{23}\cdots \\
3.\ 0. & a_{31} & a_{32} & a_{33}\cdots \\
\cdots & \cdots & \cdots & \cdots \\
n.\ 0. & a_{n1} & a_{n2} & a_{n3}\cdots \\
\cdots & \cdots & \cdots & \cdots
\end{array}
$$

Here each a_{ij} is one of the fixed ten symbols $0, 1, 2, \ldots, 9$. subject to the conditions discussed earlier.

Cantor then argues that if there is a one-to-one correspondence between N and (0,1), then the above list is complete in the sense that each real number in (0,1) must occur once in the above list. Let us consider a number,

$b = 0.b_1b_2b_3\ldots$, where

$$b_1 = 0, \text{ if } a_{11} \neq 0, \qquad b_2 = 0 \text{ if } a_{22} \neq 0,$$
$$= 1, \text{ if } a_{11} = 0; \qquad = 1 \text{ if } a_{22} = 0;$$

In general

$$b_n = 0 \text{ if } a_{nn} \neq 0;$$
$$= 1 \text{ if } a_{nn} = 0$$

Clearly $b \in$ (0,1). But b is different from the first number in the list, for it differs at the first decimal place.... It is different from the nth number in the list, for it differs at the nth place. Thus b is different from each number in the list. Therefore, the above list is not complete. In fact, there is no way to make it complete. The set (0,1) is uncountable. Just as the cardinality of N is denoted by $\aleph_0$, that of (0,1) is denoted by $\aleph_1$. For reasons which we will soon learn, $\aleph_1$ is also denoted by the letter c. It stands for the first letter of the word continuum. Thus we proved that the cardinality of unit interval (0,1) is c.

3.8.2 Cardinality of Points on Unit Line Segment

We know that real numbers can be represented by points on an infinitely extended line, called the real line. This establishes a one-to-one correspondence between the set of real numbers and points on a line. If we restrict our attention to the correspondence between the real numbers in the open unit interval (0,1) and an open line segment of unit length, then it follows that the cardinality of the open unit line segment is c.

At this point it may be interesting to note that the addition or deletion of countably many elements (finitely many included) does not change the cardinality of an uncountable set. In particular, the cardinality of points in an open segment AB (where points A and B are excluded) and in a closed segment AB (where points A and B are included) is the same.

3.8.3 Cardinality of Points on a Line Segment of any Length

As seen in Section 3.6.3, points on the line segment AB are in one-to-one correspondance with the points on the line segment CD; even though the

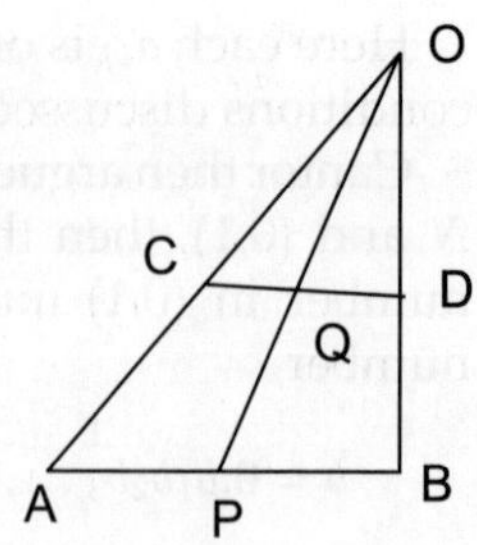

two line segments are of different lengths. Therefore it is clear that the cardinality of any line segment is the same.

Since the cardinality of a unit line segment is c, the cardinality of a line segment of any length, be it one centimetre or one kilometre, is c.

This fact resolves the paradox of 2500 years standing. Achilles does not cross more points in order to overtake the tortoise.

3.8.4 Cardinality of Points on a Line

It is intuitively clear that there is a one-to-one correspondence between points on an open line segment AB and an open semi-circular arc ACB of the same length. Therefore the cardinality of points on the semi-circular arc is c. Let ACB touch a line L at C. L is extended both ways as an infinite line, and C is chosen to be equidistant from A and B. From the centre O of the semi-circle, a variable ray cuts the line at the variable point P and the semi-circle at the variable point Q. Clearly the pairs P, Q of points so obtained establish a one-to-one correspondence between the open arc ACB and the infinite line L. This shows that the cardinality of an infinitely extended line is c. The real line is called a continuum. This is why its cardinality is denoted by c. It then follows that the cardinality of the set R of real numbers is c, as there is one-to-one correspondence between the points on a line and real numbers.

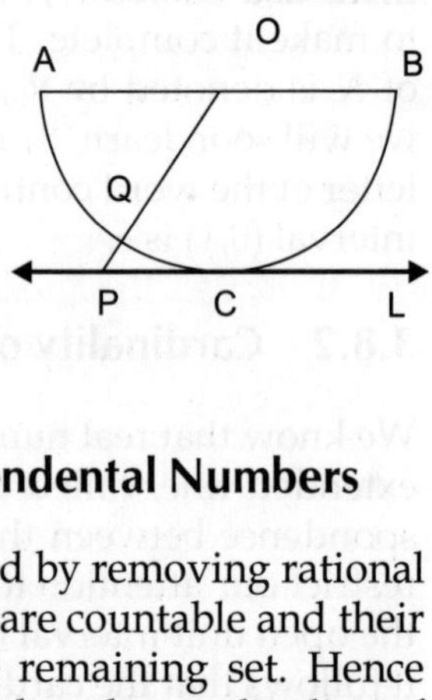

3.8.5 Cardinality of Irrational and Transcendental Numbers

Let I be the set of irrational numbers. I is obtained by removing rational numbers from R. But we have seen that rationals are countable and their removal does not change the cardinality of the remaining set. Hence the cardinality of I is c. Similarly it is known that the cardinality of transcendental numbers is c, though very few of them are explicitly known.

The following story highlights how uncountably many "irrationals" create serious problems for countable rationals in an unknown university, which may resemble many Indian universities.

3.9 A Story of an Exam in a University of Reals

This is a story of a fictitious university. If it resembles in reality any Indian university, it is merely a coincidence. Although the story is not real, the characters in the story are reals (i.e. real numbers). All the students in the university are real numbers—rational as well as irrational. Rationals were countable but irrationals were uncountable. Rationals, true to their name, were quite reasonable. Naturals, among them, were very regular in class. Integers also were quite disciplined. They very well knew where to sit in class and how to behave. Rationals had some problems initially. But later they could be taught to move in an orderly manner, like naturals.

But irrationals were rowdies. Algebraic among them were somehow manageable. But transcendentals created a big problem. Though unaccountably many, they were hardly seen in class. Occasionally a few of them like $\pi, e, 2^{\sqrt{2}}$ and their friends could be located in class.

The new vice-chancellor of the university was a real academician. He made the examination system more rational so that only deserving students could get through. The result was obvious. Only rationals passed the examinations and all the irrationals failed. Comparing the (cardinal) number of successful students with that of failures, it was natural to conclude that the rate of passing was zero per cent.

The next day's headlines in the local newspapers were quite devastating: "Student's Massacre in University of Reals". "Antistudent policies of insensitive VC". "Remove VC", the Enemy of Students". Some journalists even suspected nepotism. Since the examiners were rational, they favoured the rational numbers.

There was a big pandemonium in the campus. General elections were round the corner. So the vice-chancellor was removed and a more docile, more obliging person was appointed as the new vice-chancellor. The new VC removed all rational examiners. As a result, in the next examinations all the irrationals got through the examinations and all the rationals failed.

But the irrationals' joy was short-lived. Very soon they realised that it was not enough to get through the exams. They must have a certificate of passing. In fact some irrationals felt that the certificate was more important than success in the examinations.

Students formed a queue before the window through which they were supposed to get the certificates. But only countably many could stand in the queue. So they decided to join the convocation procession any way. They thought that since a procession consists of infinitely long rows of infinitely many columns, all of them could easily be accomodated in the procession. But to their dismay, the procession could absorb only countably many aspirants.

Thus the change in VC did not solve the problems of the irrationals.

It has been learnt that the irrationals have joined politics. For this is probably the only profession where you do not need any formal qualification.

3.10 Infinity of Infinities

Let us order the cardinal numbers. We will say that the cardinal number of a set X is less than that of a set Y, if there is a one-to-one correspondence between X and a subset of Y but not vice versa. If X and Y are finite sets with m and n elements respectively, then the cardinal number of X is less than that of Y if and only if $m < n$. The first infinite cardinal number is that of N, which is obviously greater than any finite cardinal. We have seen that the cardinality of (0,1) and hence of R is strictly greater than that of N. For this reason, we have $0 < 1 < 2 < \ldots\ldots < \aleph_0 < c$.

It is only natural to ask – is there any set of cardinality greater than c? The answer is yes. It can be proved that the set of all subsets of R is such a set. In fact if X is any set, finite or infinite and Y is the set of all subsets of X, then the cardinality of Y is strictly greater than that of X.

If X has no element, i.e., if $X = \Phi$, then $Y = \{\Phi\}$ and thus cardinality of Y is 1. If X has two elements say $\{1, 2\}$, then Y has 4 elements, $Y = \{\phi, \{1\}, \{2\}, \{1, 2\}\}$. In general, if X has n elements then Y has 2^n elements. For this reason, if the cardinality of X is $|X|$, where X is finite or infinite, that of Y is denoted by $2^{|x|}$. In this notation we have an infinite chain of cardinalities.

$$0 < 1 < 2 < \ldots < \aleph_0 < c < 2^c < 2c < 2^{c^c} < \ldots.$$

We know that there cannot be a fractional cardinality, i.e., there is no set of cardinality, say $3\frac{1}{2}$ For this reason if X and Y are two sets of cardinalities, n and $n + 1$, there is no set of cardinality strictly greater than that of X and strictly less than that of Y. Can we make a similar statement, when X and Y are infinite? It can be proved that $2^{\aleph_0} = c$ i.e. the cardinality of R and that of the set of all subsets of N is the same. Between n and 2^n, there are many sets of different cardinalities (How many?). So it is natural to expect infinite cardinal numbers between $|X|$ and $2^{|x|}$, when X is infinite. But as Cantor himself has conclusively proved, the rules of finite numbers cannot be straightway extended to infinite cases. Cantor thought that there was no cardinal number lying between $\aleph_0$ and c. This is known as Cantor's continuum hypothesis. More generally, if X is infinite, then by the axiom there is no set of cardinal numbers strictly lying between $|X|$ and $2^{|X|}$ – this is called Cantor's generalised continuum hypothesis. In 1931, Kurt Godel proved that the continuum hypothesis cannot be proved by using other axioms of set theory. In 1965, P J Cohen proved that Cantor's hypothesis can be replaced by its negation without disturbing other axioms of set theory. Both Godel and Cohen got the highest mathematics awards for their results. Thus we now have two set theories, one having the continuum hypothesis as one of its axioms and the one which has the negation of the continuum hypothesis as one of the axioms.

Conclusion

The concept of set and one-to-one correspondence put the notion of infinity into proper perspective. It resolved long standing paradoxes and gave mathematics a tremendous versatility so that it could be used in almost all branches of knowledge. References 1 to 9 give additional information.

Lecture 4

Paradise Lost, Paradise Regained

Abstract

In this lecture, we will see how paradoxes occured in even the intuitive set theory of Cantor and how these paradoxes can be avoided by some ingenious devices. The axioms proposed in the Zermelo–Fraenkel set theory are listed at the end of the lecture as an appendix.

4.1 Introduction

The German mathematician, David Hilbert (1862–1943) described Cantor's set theory as a mathematician's paradise, primarily for three reasons. One is that it helps to give a precise definition for infinity, which had been evading mathematicians for thousands of years and creating all sorts of logical problems in the development of mathematics. More importantly, it is the single concept on which the whole edifice of mathematics remains erect. Thirdly, it liberated mathematics from the bonds of real numbers and thus increased its reach and utility.

Cantor's paradise would have remained a solid structure if its set theoretic foundation remained sound i.e., if the concept of set would have remained free from contradictions. But at the beginning of the twentieth century it became amply clear that Cantor's concept of a set was not as secure as it appeared to be initially. But since it was repeatedly demonstrated that the set theory was useful in several ways, mathematicians were not ready to discard it easily. Instead, they used many ingenious methods to remove the drawbacks and restore the set theory to its privileged position in mathematics.

In this lecture we will have a look at the difficulties in accepting the set theory of Cantor and see how mathematicians removed these difficulties.

4.2 Cracks in the Foundation of Paradise

We have seen that every set has a cardinal number attached to it. For a finite set it is a natural number, the so-called number of elements in it. For infinite sets, we have a chain of cardinal numbers starting from $\aleph_0$. This raises a natural question. What is the cardinal number for the set S if it is the set of all the sets which we can think of. Clearly S is a set with the largest cardinality in the sense that no set has cardinality greater than that of S. But how can this happen? This was a question raised by Cantor himself in the year 1895. For he had proved that if X is a set, the cardinality of the set of all subsets of X is strictly greater than the cardinality of X. Therefore, the cardinality of the set of all subsets of S has to be greater than the cardinality of S. But the cardinality of S is the greatest! How can there be anything greater than the greatest?

He faced a similar problem with ordinal numbers. The problem is known as the Burali Forti paradox. Since it is a bit technical in nature, we will refrain from stating it here.

However, the paradox that Bertrand Russell faced is more celebrated. Therefore we will discuss it in more detail. The story dates back to the year 1902. German mathematician Gottlob Frege was then on the verge of completing a two-volume treatise on the foundation of arithmetics. The first volume was already published in 1893. The manuscript of the second volume had already gone to press. When Gottlob Frege received a post card from " a young lecturer Mr. Bertrand Russell ", he had completed writing the preface to the second volume. He had been working on this project for over twelve years. But there was little else he could do than add the following sentence as a post script to his work: " A scientist can hardly meet with anything more undesirable than to have the foundation give way just as the work is finished. A letter from Mr. Bertrand Russell put me in this position at the moment the work was nearly through the press ".

What was so explosive in this letter, that the foundation so meticulously constructed for twelve long years, was immediately blown to pieces? In order to understand this clearly, we begin with the definition of a set as, proposed by Cantor.

DEFINITION: A set is a collection into a whole, of definite, separate objects of one's intuition or thought.

The above definition gives us complete freedom to construct any set that we can think of. A set of natural numbers, a set of ideas, a set of flowers, the set of all objects describable in exactly eleven English words, are all legitimate sets according to the above definition. The set N of natural numbers is not a natural number. Thus N is not a member of itself. In symbols, $N \notin N$. On the other hand, the set of ideas I is an idea. Hence I is a member of itself ($I \in I$). Similarly, the set F of flowers is not a member of itself ($F \notin F$). But the set O of all objects describable in exactly eleven English words is a member of itself ($O \in O$). Thus there are some sets which contain themselves as elements and some sets which do not contain themselves as elements. Let us call the sets which do not contain themselves as members, as normal sets. The sets which contain themselves as members may then be called abnormal sets. Since abnormal sets look problematic, we will concentrate our attention on normal sets. Suppose N is the set of all normal sets. An immediate natural question then is, "Is N normal or abnormal?" This was precisely the question asked by Russell to Frege.

If N is normal, then since it contains all normal sets, we have $N \in N$. But this makes it abnormal. On the other hand, if N is abnormal, then it will be an element of N i.e. $N \in N$. But this makes N normal. Thus either way, we are led to a contradiction.

The popular version of Russell's paradox is the well-known Barber's paradox.

4.3 Barber's Dilemma: To Shave or not to Shave

In a village, there was a barber. He was the only barber in the village. It happened once that a journalist wanted to interview the barber. So he went to the village and expressed his intention to the very first person he met. By chance, he was the village barber himself.

"I want to meet the village barber", said the journalist.

The barber was in a jocular mood.

"I understand your word 'village'. But what is a 'barber"'?, he asked!

"You do not know what a 'barber' is?", the journalist asked, making efforts to keep his cool. "A barber is a person who shaves precisely those who do not shave themselves. Do you know anybody like this?", the journalist asked.

The barber remained lost in thought and finally replied, "Am I supposed to shave or not to shave myself? Either way I am in trouble. If I shave myself, I am violating the definition of a barber. For I am supposed to shave only those who do not shave themselves. If I do not shave myself, there is still a problem. For I am supposed to shave everybody, that includes me too, who does not shave oneself".

Russell's paradox was a serious blow to the logical soundness of the set theory initiated by Cantor. The very definition of the term "set" seemed to be faulty. And on faulty notion we cannot construct a sound theory. The paradise seemed to have been lost!

Usually, when such contradictions are noticed, the natural reaction is to abandon the theory. Mathematicians of earlier days were reluctant to deal with actual infinity precisely for this reason. But by the year 1902, the set theory had shown promises not only to solve many long-standing problems but also to play a central role in unifying the whole mathematics. In the words of David Hilbert, the set theory is probably the greatest achievement which our age can boast of. Therefore attempts were made to save the set theory, or at least as much useful part of the set theory as possible. There are several such attempts. We will discuss here a solution offered by Zermelo, which is widely used by the mathematical community.

4.4 Can Everything be Defined?

The German mathematician, Ernst Zermelo's answer to Russell's paradox was axiomatisation of mathematics. He put forward his scheme when a great change was taking place in the meaning of mathematical truth. The existence of more than one geometries, all contradicting each other and all equally true, was creating a revolution in the philosophy of mathematics. It was in this atmosphere that Zermelo presented his solution to the problems created by Russell's paradox. The central idea of the solution was that everything could not be defined. Euclid in his book on geometry began with 23 definitions of the terms he would use in the succeeding part of his book. For example, he defined " A point is one which has no parts ". If this was to be accepted as a definition of the term " point ", then one must define " part ". Thus a meaningful definition of the word " point " demanded meaningful definition of the word " part ". If we dared to define " A part is one which is not whole ", then the immediate question would have been about the definition of " whole ", and this search for definitions would be never ending. In general if X_0 was to be " precisely " defined then we would require a chain of definition of terms $X_1, X_2, \dots X_n, \dots$. Moreover, for the logical soundness of the definition of the term X_n, we could not have used the terms $X_0, X_1, \dots X_{n-1}$ in the definition. If we assume that our vocabulary is finite, then we would have to come back to X_0 at some stage, which is logically incorrect. Otherwise we would have an infinite chain of definitions. But it is beyond the comprehension of us mortals to deal with infinitely many definitions. Therefore, since it is unavoidable, we accept some terms as basic or primitive. They have no definition. For similar reasons, we will have to accept some statements as true statements without demanding a proof of their validity. They are called axioms or postulates. Zermelo accepted " set " as an undefined term. He realised that the main culprit in Russell's paradox was the definition of a set given by Cantor. The definition allowed any collection of objects that we could thinsk of as a set. So he proposed to accept set as a primitive term, and to choose axioms in such a way that while all important results in mathematics could be retained, the problematic sets, like Russell's sets, remain outside the purview of mathematics. His scheme is called the axiomatic set theory as against the naive set theory of Cantor.

4.5 Paradise Regained

Zermelo noticed that when we begin the study of a particular field of knowledge, we are interested in the objects of that field only. One may call it the world of cognition or the universal set. To form a set of objects of our choice, we then select objects from this universal set, using some fixed criteria. For example, if we intent to study real solutions to some equations, we pick up elements from the set of real numbers using the criterion that these real numbers satisfy the given system of equations. The set of real numbers is now our universe of cognition or the universal set from which the objects are to be selected to form the set. The system of equations offers the criterion for selection. If a real number satisfies the equation, it becomes a member of the set, otherwise it is not.

He then " legalises " his scheme by accepting the following proposition as an axiom. The axiom is called the axiom of selection.

4.5.1 Axiom of Selection

Let U be a set. Let $P(x)$ be a statement which is meaningful for every object in U. By meaningful, we mean it is either true or false but not undecidable. Then there exists a set which consists of exactly those elements x in U for which $P(x)$ is a true statement. Now the axiom of selection disallows the problematic set $\{A|A \notin A\}$ in Zermelo's scheme. The nearest that we can have is the set $\{A \in U|A \notin A\}$. This small difference, which has big philosophical implications, removes the logical difficulties of mathematicians. For now we can legitimately claim that the set $S = \{A \in U|A \notin A\}$ does not exist, in the sense that it is outside U and hence outside our purview. In other words, we have the following theorem.

THEOREM: The set $S = \{A \in U|A \notin A\}$ is outside U. l

PROOF: Clearly there are only two possibilities: either $S \in S$ or $S \notin S$.

But the option $S \in S$ is impossible. For $S \in S$ leads to the contradictory result that $S \notin S$.

Therefore our first assertion is that $S \notin S$.

If $S \in U$, then together with $S \notin S$ it implies that $S \in S$. But this is contradictory to the result that $S \notin S$. Hence $S \notin U$.

4.5.2 Wolf Inside Compound

In Zermelo's scheme of set theory, the known paradox is kept outside the periphery of mathematics. In the process, he definitely keeps the essential results of mathematics undisturbed. But essentially he has not resolved the paradox, he has only avoided it by a brilliant device. Russell's paradox appeared after a lapse of 27 years. Can anybody say with confidence that some other paradox will not appear after a lapse of 270 years? One of the great mathematicians of his time, Henri Poincaré compared Zermelos's device with the behaviour of a shepherd who wanted to protect his sheep by raising a compound around them. The shepherd put the fence so that a wolf outside the fence would not enter and kill the sheep. But he does not know whether there is a wolf inside the compound already. And there was a wolf inside the compound so meticulously raised by Zermelo. The name of the wolf was Berry's paradox.

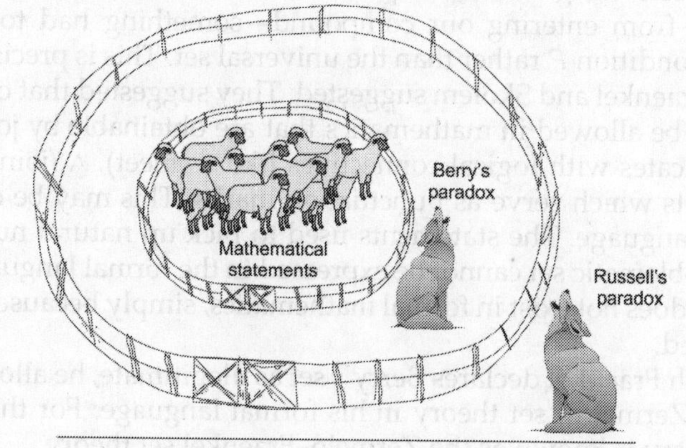

Berry's paradox is about a set of natural numbers N. The elements of N can be described in several ways. For example, ninety nine may be unambiguously described as the greatest two-digit integer. Equally unambiguously, it is the smallest natural number greater than ninety eight. "Three times thirty three" is yet another description of ninety nine. N has one more interesting property. Its every non-empty subset has the smallest element. This is not true for every subset of real numbers. For example, the unit open interval (0,1) has no smallest element. With this much preparation, let us understand the question raised by Berry.

4.5.3 Berry's Paradox

Let S be the set of all natural numbers expressible in less than fifty English words. Let T be the set of all natural numbers which are not in S. Let a be the smallest natural number in T. Berry's question is "Is a in S"?

Clearly this question can have only one answer, either $a \in S$ or $a \notin S$. It cannot be both.

Now since T consists of elements which are not in S and $a \in T$, it is natural to conclude that $a \notin S$. On the other hand, since a can be unambiguously described in less than fifty English words as "the smallest element of T", it certainly lies in S.

Berry's troublesome set may be expressed in symbols as $S = \{x \in N | P(x)\}$, where $P(x)$ stands for a statement that x is expressible in less than fifty words of the English language.

The set S described before follows Zermelo's dictum. It is constructed by selecting elements from the universal set N according to the rule $P(x)$ which is explicitly stated. Moreover the universal set N used in the construction of S occurs too frequently to avoid in mathematics. Therefore, following the footsteps of Zermelo, if we want to prohibit Berry's set from entering our compound – something had to be done about the condition P rather than the universal set. This is precisely what logicians Fraenkel and Skolem suggested. They suggested that only those statements be allowed in mathematics that are obtainable by joining the basic predicates with logical connectives like $\vee$ (meet), $\wedge$ (join), $\sim$ (not) and brackets which serve as punctuation marks. This may be described as formal language. The statements used to pick up natural numbers in Berry's problematic set cannot be expressed in the formal language. Thus Berry's set does not exist in formal mathematics, simply because it cannot be expressed.

Although Fraenkel declares Berry's set as illegitimate, he allows all the axioms of Zermelo's set theory in his formal language. For this reason, this set theory is known as the Zermelo–Fraenkel set theory.

The paradise built by Cantor and lost due to paradoxes was regained by Zermelo and Fraenkel. Of course, there were several others who contributed to the conquest but this volume is too short to describe their contributions.

The axioms of the Zermelo–Fraenkel set theory are listed at the end of this lecture.

Conclusion

Cantor resolved old paradoxes related to the concept of infinity. But in course of time, paradoxes were noticed in his theory also. These paradoxes have been avoided – although not resolved – by some ingenious methods. But no fool-proof method could be evolved which would guarantee freedom from contradiction.

In fact we are now coming to the conclusion that we may never be able to give such a guarantee. The only solace for mathematicians is that no paradox has been noticed in the last ninety years. The references given in the end can help students learn much more about the basics of mathematical literature.

Appendix

Symbols

$\forall$ For all	$\Leftrightarrow$ iff	$\in$ is an element of
$\exists$ there exists	$\vee$ or	$=$ equal to
$\exists\,!$ there exists unique	$\wedge$ and	$\neq$ not equal to
$\cup$ Union	$\sim$ not	Φ the empty set
$\Rightarrow$ implies	$\subseteq$ is a subset of	
iff if and only if		

Axioms of Set Theory

1. **Axiom of extensionality:**

$$\{\forall\, x, y\, (\forall z\, (z \in x \Leftrightarrow z \in y) \Rightarrow x = y)\}.$$

Two sets are equal iff they have the same members.

2. **Axiom of null set:**

$$\exists\, x\, \forall\, y\, (\sim y \in x).$$

There exists a set with no elements

3. **Axiom of ordered pairs:**

$$\forall\, x,\; y\, \exists\, z\, \forall\, w\, (w \in z \Leftrightarrow w = x \vee w = y).$$

If x and y are sets, then the unordered pair $\{x, y\}$ is also a set.

4. **Axiom of union of sets:**

$$\forall\, x\, \exists\, y\, \forall\, z\, (z \in y \Leftrightarrow \exists\, t(z \in t \wedge t \in x)$$

The union of sets is a set.

5. **Axiom of infinity:**

$$\exists\, x\, (\Phi \in x \wedge \forall\, y\, (y \in x \Rightarrow y \cup \{y\} \in x)$$

There exists a set x such that it contains the empty set, and such that if y is a member of x then $y \cup \{y\}$ is also a member of x. This axiom guarantees the infinite set (The axiom is crucial as one cannot experience infinity).

6. **Axiom of replacement:**

$$\forall\, t_1, \ldots, t_k\, (\forall\, x\, \exists\,!\, y\, (A_n\, (x, y, t_1 \ldots, \ldots t_k)) \Rightarrow \forall\, u\, \exists\, B(u, v),$$

where $B(u, v) \equiv \forall r(r \in \theta \Leftrightarrow \exists\, s(s \in u \wedge A_n(s, r, t_1 \ldots, t_k))$

This axiom is difficult to write in the natural language. It is actually a family of n axioms and roughly says that any property that can be stated in the formal language can be used to define a set. This avoids Berry's problematic set.

7. **Power set axiom:**

$$\forall\, x\, \exists\, y\, \forall\, z\, (z \in y \Leftrightarrow z \subseteq x).$$

There exists for each x, the set y of all subsets of x (this enables us to construct a set of higher cardinality).

8. **Axiom of choice:**

If $a \to A_a \neq \Phi$ is a function defined for all $a \in X$ then $\exists$ another function $f(a)$ for $a \in X$, and $f(a) \in A_a$ (This axiom allows us to do an infinite amount of choosing, even though we have no property that would define the choice function and thus enable us to use Axiom 6).

9. **Axiom of regularity:**

$$\forall\, x\, \exists\, y\, (x = \Phi \vee (y \in x \wedge \forall\, z(z \in y \Rightarrow z \notin x)).$$

This axiom explicitly prohibits $x \in x$ (This avoids Russell's paradox).

Lecture 5

Concerns of a Mathematician

Abstract

When one learns or teaches different branches or subjects of mathematics, we find that there are certain underlying features that are common to all of them. It is important that one recognises these features in order to understand mathematics as a whole. They are presented here as concerns, the appreciation of which will help everybody enhance and enrich one's holistic outlook towards the whole gamut of mathematics.

5.1 Introduction

In this lecture, we use the word "mathematician" in a wide sense. Anybody who genuinely loves and therefore studies the subject of mathematics and obtains some competency in it, is a mathematician for our purpose here. Such a person may be a student, or a teacher (in a school, college or university) or a researcher. He or she may also be engaged in any other profession but show real interest, some understanding and appreciation of mathematics though he/she may not actually be an expert, by any standard, in any part of mathematics. We would like to bring out here what, according to us, such mathematicians should be concerned with. If they are students, they should be in a position to understand and appreciate the concerns that we are putting forward here for their progress in the study of mathematics. If they are teachers or researchers, they should be able to pass on these concerns through their talks and writings, to their listeners and readers. We now enumerate, with some examples and explanations, these concerns that we expect a mathematician to know and display in his/her work.

5.2 Mathematics can be done in Multiple Ways

Let us prove this statement with examples. One of the simplest example is that of finding HCF. HCF of two given natural numbers can be found by finding the prime factors of each of them and then obtaining the product of those prime factors which are common to both the given natural numbers. Alternatively, HCF can be found by using Euclid's algorithm. The two methods are different in nature – Euclid's algorithm is more suitable for computers and hence is finding its place in present-day textbooks. Traditional textbooks of even a few generations back only explain the method based on prime-factorisation.

The second example is that of solving the system $Ax = b$ of n linear, simultaneous, algebraic, non-homogeneous and independent equations. Here x is an $n \times 1$ vector of n unknowns, A is an $n \times n$ non-singular matrix of coefficients of the unknowns, and b is an $n \times 1$ non-null vector, elements of A and b being known. Now this system can be solved, i.e., values of x can be found by various methods like the Cramer's rule, Gaussian elimination, and the Gauss–Jordan method. Solving using Cramer's rule is very important for theoretical development, but it is not a polynomial–time algorithm, while Gaussian elimination and the Gauss–Jordan method are polynomial–time algorithms.

Another example is that of solving a linear programming problem – three methods, namely those given by Dantzig, Khachian and Karmarkar are available. They are completely different in their approaches, though all of them are iterative methods. Dantzig's simplex method consists of moving from one corner of the feasible region of solutions, to an adjacent corner along the boundary of the feasible region. Hence it is also called an extreme point method. Khachian's ellipsoidal method is an exterior point method, as it starts, in each iteration, from a point outside the feasible region and moves finally to the solution of the problem. On the other hand, Karmarkar's method is an interior point method as it starts, in each iteration, from a point inside the feasible region and finally moves to the solution of the problem.

5.3 The Solution to a Problem in Mathematics may be None, only One, or Many

To explain this we again refer to a linear programming problem (LPP). If the constraints of an LPP are such that the feasible region (FR) is empty, then that LPP has no solution. If the line (hyperplane in general) representing a particular value of the objective function (OF) is parallel to the line corresponding to one of the constraints that binds the FR, then that LPP will have many (optimal) solutions. Otherwise, the LPP will have one and only one (i.e., unique) solution.

Let us take another example – that of simultaneous linear algebraic equations. The equations $x + y = 5$ and $2x + 2y = 12$ have no solution; the equations $x + y = 3$ and $4x + 4y = 12$ have many solutions, while the equations $x + y = 3$ and $2x + 3y = 8$ have one and only one solution.

Many problems in recreational mathematics can be formulated by Diophantine equations and they have, many times, more than one solution. As an example, we leave it to the reader to find the solution to the following problem: Distribute Rs. 100/- using exactly 50 currency notes having denominations of Rs. 50, 20, 10, 5 and 1 only. This problem has more than one solution.

5.4 Some Situations in Mathematics are Unsolved

Again many examples can be given. To whet your appetite, we shall relate a few. Goldbach's conjecture, posed in 1742, states: Every even integer greater then 4 can be expressed as a sum of two odd primes. Though this conjecture is verified to be true for many even integers (the verification being comparatively easy now with the availability of computers), we do not have a mathematical proof of the validity of the statement of the conjecture and hence this conjecture is an example of an unsolved (i.e., open) problem in mathematics. Another example is the question about Mersenne numbers – numbers of the form $2^n - 1$, $n = 1, 2, 3 \ldots$ (see Lecture 10, Section 10.12). Determining which Mersenne numbers are prime and which are not, is unresolved till today.

5.5 Some Situations in Mathematics can be Shown to be Unsolvable

For example, it has been proved that one cannot give a procedure of trisecting a given angle using a compass and a straight edge only. One can trisect angles of some special measure (e.g., a right angle) using the compass and straight edge but a general procedure for any arbitrary angle cannot be given, i.e., even in the future, it will be impossible to come up with such a procedure. Such results are negative in nature, in the sense, that they state what cannot be done under the given conditions. These results, and of course their proofs are landmarks in the history of mathematics.

Another such impossibility result is that there is no algebraic formula to express the roots of a general polynomial of degree 5 or more (similar to the well-known quadratic formula for polynomials of degree 2).

5.6 Pictures Drawn to Solve Mathematical Problems can be Deceptive

We first cite, to illustrate this statement, the famous proof of the fact that any given triangle is isosceles.

Consider any △ ABC. Let the perpendicular bisector of BC and the bisector of ∠ A meet at D. (Depending on whether they meet inside or outside △ ABC, we have Fig. 5.1 and Fig. 5.2 respectively). Drop perpendiculars on AB and AC from D.

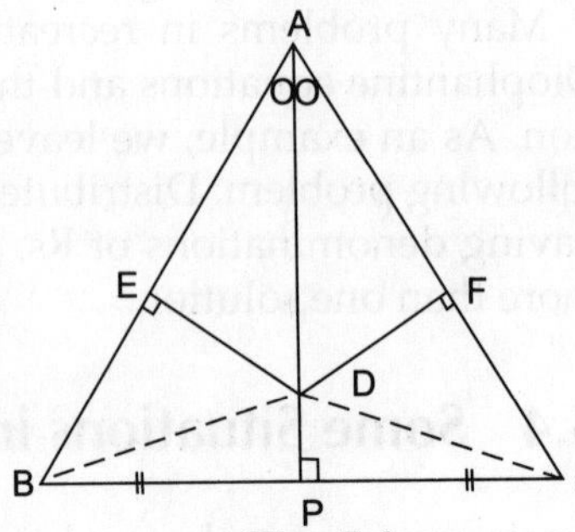

Fig. 5.1

Now △ AED ≅ △ AFD (as ∠ EAD = ∠ FAD, ∠ AED = ∠ AFD = 90° and AD is common, by the use of the ASA principle the two triangles are congruent).

Hence ED = FD and AE = AF (1)

Then △ EBD ≅ △ FCD (as the two △s are right △s, ED = FD and BD = CD since D lies on the ⊥ bisector of BC)

Hence EB = FC (2)

In the case of Fig. 5.1, adding (1) and (2) and in the case of Fig. 5.2, subtracting (2) from (1), we get AB = AC, proving that △ ABC is isosceles.

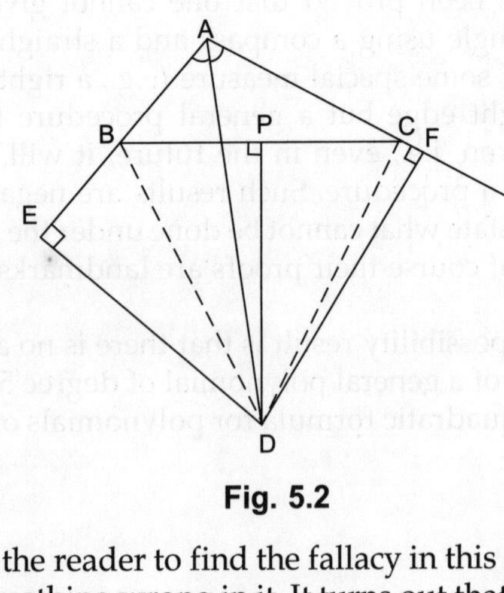

Fig. 5.2

We leave it to the reader to find the fallacy in this proof. It is clear that there must be something wrong in it. It turns out that Figs. 5.1 and 5.2 are deceptive. The reader should find out, by arguing out logically (and not just by drawing the right figure using the instruments of a geometry box) the right figure representing the construction designed above, to prove the statement.

Consider another example: ABCD is a trapezium with AB = 2 units, BC = 10 units, AD = 8 units. M is the mid-point of AD and MC bisects the angle BCD. Find the area of the trapezium. See whether you can draw the correct figure that will represent the description of the trapezium in the beginning itself. Solve the problem and then try to find out if there is any deception in the figure that you drew at the start.

5.7 Mathematical Facts have Analogies in Other Fields of Knowledge

Any natural number can be expressed as a product of its prime factors. For example, $360 = 2 \times 2 \times 2 \times 3 \times 3 \times 5$. For any natural number, its prime factors become its, so to say, building blocks. Similarly, in chemistry, any compound can be expressed using its building blocks viz., the natural elements of the periodic table. For example, water = H_2O, sulphuric acid = H_2SO_4. Following this analogy in chemistry, one can write 360 as $360 = 2_3 3_2 5_1$, although it is customary in mathematics to write it as $360 = 2^3 3^2 5$.

There is something more to this analogy. The way of expressing a natural number using its prime factors is unique. Similarly, we know that a compound in chemistry can be expressed in terms of its natural elements in one and only one way. Thus, there is an anology between the fundamental theorem of arithmetic (stated in Lecture 10, Section 10.9) on one hand, and the process of expressing a chemical compound in terms of the natural elements of the periodic table, on the other.

We would like to point out further that no analogy is fully complete either in mathematics or in any other field. The analogy between a tree (giving shelter to anybody, good or bad) and a *sthitapradnya* person described in the *Bhagavat Gita* (treating joy and grief, hot and cold etc, on the same footing) is not complete, because a tree cannot walk but the person can. Similarly, the chemical analogy described in the paragraph above, is not complete. This is so because the building blocks (viz. primes) of natural numbers are infinite, while those of a chemical compound (viz natural elements of the periodic table in chemistry) are finite in number.

Another analogy is worth mentioning. The theorem of total probability states that if $\{B_1, B_2, \ldots B_n\}$ is a partition of sample space S, and A is any event in S, then.

$$P(A) = \sum_{i=1}^{n} P(B_i)P(A|B_i).$$

This formula is very much analogous to the formula

$$C(A) = \sum_{i=1}^{n} V(B_i)C(A|B_i).$$

where $C(A|B_i)(i = 1, 2, .3 \ldots)$ is the concentration of a dissolvable substance A in the volume $V(B_i)$ of water, with $\sum_{i=1}^{n} V(B_i) = 1$. The second formula gives the concentration $C(A)$ of A when the water in all the n beakers is collected in one container.

Note that in the first formula $\sum_{i=1}^{n} P(B_i) = 1$. This analogy is also, as expected, not complete since $P(B_i)$ is dimensionless, i.e., a pure number, while $V(B_i)$ has the dimensions of volume. The same is true with $P(A)$ and $P(A|B_i)$ on one hand, and $C(A)$ and $C(A|B_i)$ on the other.

5.8 Mathematics has a Recreational Aspect

There are plenty of puzzles and riddles, the reading and studying of which gives us a lot of enjoyment. The recreational aspect of mathematics is considered so important that there is a separate journal – *Journal of Recreational Mathematics* – devoted to this aspect.

We give one illustration of this aspect here. You may be aware of magic squares. We give here a different kind of magic square which provides recreation and therefore enjoyment. See in Fig. 5.3, a 4×4 magic square, each square of which is either shaded or unshaded. Further, each square has a number as well as a letter in it. The magic of this square is as follows: Choose the number from any square. Spell out that number. You will find every letter of that spelling somewhere in the square. If the letter is in an unshaded square, take the number of that square with positive sign; if the letter is in a shaded square, take the number of that square with negative sign. Find the sum of the numbers corresponding to all the letters in the spelling of the chosen number taking the numbers with proper signs as explained above. You will be surprised to see that this sum is equal to the number chosen to start with. For example.

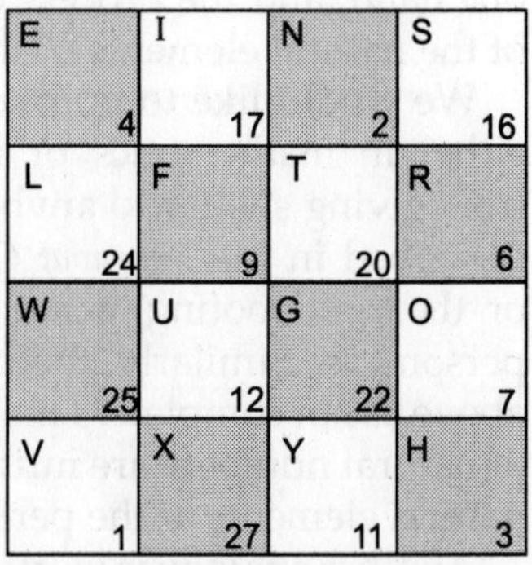
E 4
I 17
N 2
S 16
L 24
F 9
T 20
R 6
W 25
U 12
G 22
O 7
V 1
X 27
Y 11
H 3

Fig. 5.3

$$22 \rightarrow \text{Twenty two} \rightarrow 20 - 25 - 4 - 2 + 20 + 11 + 20 - 25 + 7 = 22.$$

This magic square is known as Sallow's square. Now it will be a good exercise for the reader to find other numbers (not in the square) which also have this property.

5.9 Mathematics Occurs in Every Day Life

Our day-to-day life is full of the use of technological gadgets like radio, television, computers, air conditioners, washing machines, vacuum cleaners, etc., the working of which is based on the knowledge of various fields of science. All sciences make plenty of use of mathematics. That is why, though mathematics is known as the queen of science from ancient times onwards, many people prefer to call it the servant of science. To cite mundane examples in everyday use, consider the shortcuts that we take while walking or driving. They are the straightforward applications of the theorem in plane Euclidean geometry, viz., the sum of two sides of a triangle is always greater than the third. While getting down from a slowly moving bus or train (which many people in big crowded cities have to do as buses and trains there halt for a very very short time at various stops), one must face the direction in which the bus/train is moving; otherwise one may fall. This observation is based on the concept of relative velocity from applied mathematics. Calculation of timings of solar or lunar eclipses is based on mathematics. Trajectories and paths followed by satellites, missiles etc., are calculated using mathematics. Physical and chemical reactions are governed by mathematical equations and formulas. We look into a mirror every day. We notice that the left eye or left ear is seen there on the right. This is also based on mathematical principles.

5.10 Experimentation is Extremely Important in Mathematics

Before formally teaching the theorems in plane Euclidean geometry, a good teacher asks the students to draw various triangles of different sizes, measure the angles of each of them and add up these measures, for each triangle drawn. In my student days, the year before we were taught geometry theorems, my teacher announced an attractive prize to anybody in our class who could draw a triangle, the sum of whose angles would be 200°. Similarly, in an algebra class, a teacher could ask the students to try to find positive integers x, y, z, n, satisfying the equation $x^n + y^n = z^n$, when $n \geq 3$ or simply find positive integers x, y, z such that $x^3 + y^3 = z^3$. Experimentation like this keeps students bubbling with enthusiasm by triggering their imagination, making learning challenging and appealing, teaching interesting and preparing students for things that will appear in their studies in the near future in more abstract ways.

With the availability of computers and proper software, it has become easier now to adopt experimentation in education.

5.11 Historical Aspects Play an Important Role in Mathematics

A study of the history of any subject – knowing what and how it has happened earlier – puts the learning of that subject in proper perspective and can help to make progress in the right direction. Knowing that the Pythagoras theorem, Pell's equation etc., were known to our ancients [6] can instill in us national pride as well as keep the interest in the subject alive and fresh. Knowing that integration is not just the reverse of differentiation and that it was known and practiced prior to the days when differentiation became known; knowing that the fundamental theorem of integral calculus just beautifully connects the two processes of differentiation and integration, making it extremely easy to find the integration of some functions will interest the student immensely. There are good books for studying such historical aspects [1]. We shall give here an example of a not so widely known piece of historical fact related to number systems.

In the decimal system of numbers, we write small or big numbers using the digits $0, 1, 2, \ldots 9$ – this notation is unique for every number. In ancient Indian literature, we find that 19 digits viz. $-9, -8, \ldots, -1, 0, 1, 2, \ldots 9$ were used to represent numbers in some context. In that system known as the Mishrank system [3], only the positional values of numerals were $10^0, 10^1, 10^2, \ldots$ etc, as in the decimal system. Negative digits $-1, -2, \ldots, -9$, were represented by placing a bar over them as $\bar{1}, \bar{2}, \ldots \bar{9}$. So $3\bar{7}$ would represent $(-7) \times 10^0 + 3 \times 10^1 = 23$. Thus this system did not give a unique representation of numbers, in contrast to the usual decimal system The decimal system representation is unique because the radix (base) of the system = number of digits available to represent a number. This is violated in the ancient Indian system as there, the number of digits available = 19, while radix = 10.

5.12 It is not the Numerical Answer but an Algorithm to Solve a Mathematical Problem that Counts

If one knows or discovers what steps, followed one after another, would lead to a correct answer to a given problem, giving proper justification for each step, one has practically solved the problem. For example, if the problem is: "Find two factors, differing by 40, of the 13-digit number $N = 6256586734089$", it is sufficient to give a method as follows: let $N = xy$, x and y being positive integers such that $x - y = 40$. Knowing xy

and $x-y$, find $x+y$ using the known expression $(x+y)^2 = (x-y)^2 + 4xy$. Then to find exact values of x, y, one can perform the routine high-school exercise of solving two simple simultaneous equations $x - y = a$, and $x + y = b$ with known a, b. It is not all that important to actually give $x = 2501337$ and $y = 2501297$ as the solution to the given problem though it may serve as a drill when the problem is given to school children.

In the same vein, we state that deriving the formula: $x_1, x_2 = (-b \pm \sqrt{b^2 - 4ac})/2a$ for the two roots of the quadratic equation $ax^2 + bx + c = 0$ is more important than finding the actual numerical roots of some quadratic equation with numerical values a, b, c.

One should not misinterpret this discussion to mean that we do not at all pay importance to numerical calculations. What we say is that numerical calculations have a role to play but not as significant as finding the method to a solution.

5.13 It is not the Final Answer but the Procedure or the Approach to Solve a Problem that should have an Upper Hand in Assessments

I shall illustrate this point with a factual story – the moral of the story will bring out the point clearly. As a school student, I had a question set in my question paper; it was to find the product of two big numbers, say 11 or 12 digits long. While taking down one of the numbers, I copied one of the digits incorrectly. When my teacher valued my answer-book, he gave me 9 out of 10 marks to that answer. I asked him: "Sir, I have made a mistake in noting the question. So my answer to the concerned question is wrong. Why have you given me so much marks for my answer?". The teacher replied: "The main purpose of setting this question was to see whether you students can multiply big multi-digit integers. You have inadvertently taken down one digit of one given number wrongly. You have not done this purposely or by doing that, you have not simplified the question. Further, you have found the product correctly. So you have satisfied the purpose and intention of the question. You really deserve full marks for your answer. But you must also pay for your carelessness in noting the question; otherwise you may persist in your carelessness in your further studies, knowing that you will get full credit even though you were careless. So I have deducted one mark for that". No comments are necessary, I think to drive home the intended point.

5.14 Beliefs about Mathematics Must be Right Ones

Many people believe that mathematics is exact and mathematical statements are perfect eternal truths. Such beliefs should be in the right spirit.

If you read the discussion in Lecture 6, Section 6.3 regarding different geometries, one would know and emphasise that the results in mathematics are consistent with respect to the set of axioms chosen. So if from a set of axioms, one of them is changed to a different one, one can get a surprisingly new set of results. Thus, one must be careful about forming beliefs about mathematics.

5.15 Mathematics Requires Thinking. In Fact, Mathematics is Thinking

Here we want to emphasise that the whole of mathematics is based on deductive logic. Any statement in mathematics can be stated in the form "p implies q" which is the same thing as "if p then q" (symbolically it is written as $p \to q$ or $p \supset q$, where p and q are statements (or propositions, small or big, simple or compound). For example, the statement, "Sum of the angles of a triangle is 180°" can be stated as "if d is a triangle, then the sum of the angles of d is 180°". Thus the characteristic statement of mathematics is "if p then q".

In mathematics, one has to derive new statements from the earlier known ones using deductive logic by proper thinking. In this respect, one should be able to understand that all the following statements are equivalent:

i. p implies q,

ii. q if p,

iii. p only if q,

iv. p is sufficient condition for q,

v. q is a necessary condition for p,

vi. $\sim q$ implies $\sim p$,

vii. $\sim q$ is a sufficient condition for $\sim p$,

viii. $\sim p$ is a necessary condition for $\sim q$.

Out of these equivalent statements, "$\sim q$ implies $\sim p$" is the basis of the indirect proof (in particular, a *reductio ad absurdum* proof) in order to establish "p implies q". Indirect proofs, i.e., proofs by contradiction, occupy a very highly coveted place in mathematics and hence one who is interested in mathematics must understand and appreciate its basis thoroughly. Hardy, the apostle of proof, described proof by contradiction as "one of a mathematician's finest weapons. It is a far finer gambit than any chess gambit: a chess player may offer the sacrifice of a pawn or even a piece, but a mathematician offers the game".

All this emphasises the need for the study of deductive two-valued logic to anybody interested in mathematics, as thinking in mathematics is akin to this logic.

5.16 In Mathematics, Patterns will not Suffice to Draw Valid Conclusions

Though, as pointed out earlier, experimentation is extremely important in mathematics, one has to be cautious and careful while drawing conclusions from the experiments. Experiments unfold certain patterns at times. In practice, people accept a proposition if it is verified to be true in sufficiently large (sometime, even infinite) number of cases giving rise to a pattern. But a mathematician does not allow himself/herself to do so.

We have already seen in Section 5.4 that Goldbach's conjecture is not acceptable as a valid proposition by a mathematician even though it is verified to be true in numerous cases (in fact 50 million cases, as number theorists have decomposed all even numbers up to 100 million into the sum of two primes using computers).

As another example [2], consider the polynomial $f(n) = n^7 - 28n^6 + 322n^5 - 1960n^4 + 6769n^3 - 13132n^2 + 13069n - 5040$. It gives $f(n) = n$ for $n = 1, 2, \ldots, 7$. Looking at the pattern thrown by these consecutive 7 examples, we should not jump to the conclusion that $f(n) = n$ for any natural number n. In fact, patience will show that $f(8) = 5048$. The truth about this polynomial $f(n)$ is that it is constructed by expanding, simplifying and re-arranging the terms of the expression $n + [(n-1)(n-2)(n-3)(n-4)(n-5)(n-6)(n-7)]$ and so it is but natural for it to yield n for $f(n)$ when $n = 1, 2, \ldots, 7$. Following this trick we can use the expression $2n + [(n-1)(n-2)\ldots(n-2,000,000)]$ and simplify it to the form $g(n) = \sum_{n=0}^{2000,000} a_n x^n$ which will deceptively make people believe that $g(n) = 2n$, for all n as this is so for the first 2 million natural numbers. But obviously, such a pattern seen for even such a large number (in fact 2 million) of cases cannot make us conclude that $g(n) = 2n$ for all n.

Many examples like this can be cited. Every prime ≥ 3 (and they are infinite in number) is an odd integer. From this pattern exhibited by the infinite number of primes, we should not jump to the inference that every prime is odd. That would be wrong as we have an even prime, namely 2. Similarly, consider n-digit non-negative integers. For $n = 2, 3, \ldots T_n =$ total number of n-digit non-negative integers $= 900, \ldots 0$ (9 followed by $n-1$ zeros)$= 9 \times 10^{n-1}$. In particular, $T_2 = 90$ (viz. 10 to 99), $T_3 = 900$ (namely 100 to 999) etc. From this pattern, if one rushes to conclude that $T_1 =$ total number of one digit non-negative integers $= 9$, it will be incorrect as we have 10 (viz. $0, 1, 2, \ldots 9$) one digit non-negative integers.

The history of mathematics is rich with plenty of examples in which conclusions based on patterns thrown open by finite or infinite number of cases have shocked investigators in that these patterns did not lead to correct conclusions.

5.17 Counter-Examples Work Wonders in Mathematics

As seen earlier, numerous examples following a certain pattern do not prove a proposition in mathematics. But if we want to disprove a proposition, just one example will do. As a very simple example, consider the proposition: "If p is a prime, so is $p+2$". We can disprove this by taking a single example: $p = 7$ is prime, but $p + 2 = 9$ is not.

Sophie Germain (1776–1831) wrote to the great mathematician C F Gauss, in her letter dated February 20, 1807: "If the sum of the nth powers of any two numbers is of the form $a^2 + nb^2$, then the sum of the two numbers is also of that form". Gauss in his reply, dated April 30, 1807 gave a single counter-example to disprove her proposition. He showed that $15^{11} + 8^{11}$ is of the form $a^2 + 11b^2$, but $15 + 8$ is not of the form $c^2 + 11d^2$.

Jacques Ozanam (1640–1717) stated: "The sum of all the divisors of 2^{4n} is a prime". G W Kraft gave a counter-example of $n = 2$, showing that the sum $(1 + 2 + 4 + 8 + 16 + 32 + 64 + 128 + 256)$ of all the divisors of 2^8, viz, 511 is not a prime, since $511 = 7 \times 73$. Thus Kraft's single counter-example smashed Ozanam's statement.

The ancient Chinese believed that $2^n - 2$ is not divisible by n when n is a composite. As late as 1680, G W Leibniz (1646–1716) also made this very statement. A single counter-example, namely $n = 341$, was found in the 19th century to disprove that statement. $n = 341 = 31 \times 11$ is composite, and $2^{341} - 2$ is divisible by 341. In fact, 341 is the least value of n for which the statement fails.

A number is called deficient, perfect, or abundant according as the sum of its aliquot (i.e. proper) divisors is less than, equal to, or more than the number itself. Jordanus Nemorarius (1225–1260) stated that all abundant numbers are even. Charles de Bouvelles (1470–1533) gave a single counter-example to disprove that statement—45045 is an abundant odd number. Bachet de Méziriae (1581–1638) gave the counter-example of 945 as an odd abundant number. In fact, 945 is the smallest odd abundant number.

It used to be assumed that perfect numbers alternate between 6 and 8 in their final digit. Bouvelles also made this statement. The first five perfect numbers are 6, 28, 496, 8128, and 33550336, but the 6th perfect number 8589869056 serves as a single counter-example to demolish the statement.

In the history of mathematics, many people (even renowned ones) have put forward certain propositions and have had it refuted by somebody else (sometimes after many years) by giving just a single counter-example. These are interesting happenings indeed.

5.18 Simplicity Should be Sought in Mathematics

In mathematics, as pointed out earlier, we need to prove any proposition and not just its verification (even though that verification is done for a large number of cases), for that proposition to be called a theorem (or a lemma). Naturally, if the proof is simple, it is whole-heartedly welcome. Therefore, though the four colour theorem (a former conjecture stating that given any plane separated into regions, the regions can be coloured using no more than four colours in such a way that no two adjacent regions receive the same colour) has been proved, some mathematicians still await eagerly for a simpler proof. The same is true in the case of any other result established over time.

Let us take an example. Consider the theorem: "Sum of the first n odd natural numbers is n^2". We know that it can be proved by the technique known as principle of mathematical induction. Compare that induction proof with the following proof:

$$1+3+5+\ldots+(2n-1) = (1+2+3+\ldots+2n)-(2+4+6+\ldots+2n)$$
$$= \frac{2n(2n+1)}{2} - \frac{2n(n+1)}{2} = n^2$$

This simpler and elegant proof uses the formula for the sum of the first n natural numbers.

We have an even simpler proof, a proof without words if we look at the $n \times n$ square in Fig. 5.4 and number its cells as 1, then $1, 2, 3$, followed by $1, 2, 3, 4, 5$ etc., as shown, starting from a corner of the square. This way we see that all the n^2 cells of the figure are accounted for as a sum of $1 + 3 + 5 + \ldots + (2n-1)$ cells which is the sum of the first n odd natural numbers.

1	3	5			$2n-1$
1	2	4			*
1	2	3			*
					*
					$n+1$
1	2	3	*	*	n

Fig. 5.4

Think also about the more direct proof obtained by adding the first and the last term, the second and the last but one (i.e. second last) term etc.

This shows that we should always endeavour to get simpler and still simpler proofs of mathematical propositions.

5.19 Generalisation is the Key Word in Mathematics

A mathematician, when presented with a specific challenging problem, will try to solve it. But he/she will not be satisfied in solving that particular problem only. He tries to generalise that particular problem and attempts to solve the generalised version so that the solution to the general problem can give the solution to his particular problem, as a special case. Let us see some examples of this very important aspect of mathematics.

Consider the Konigsberg bridge problem. The river Pregel flowing through the city of Konigsberg contains two islands and seven bridges as shown in Fig. 5.5. The problem posed was to decide whether it was possible to make a tour in which each bridge is traversed exactly once and return to the starting point. The problem can be modelled as a graph, having 4 vertices and 7 edges as shown in Fig. 5.6. The problem posed above is the same as finding whether this graph can be traversed in such a way that every edge is covered exactly once and one returns to the starting point of the travel. Naturally the problem was generalised to find such a tour for any graph having any number of vertices, and any number of edges, and was solved (Euler found the types of graphs for which such tours are not possible and he proved that result).

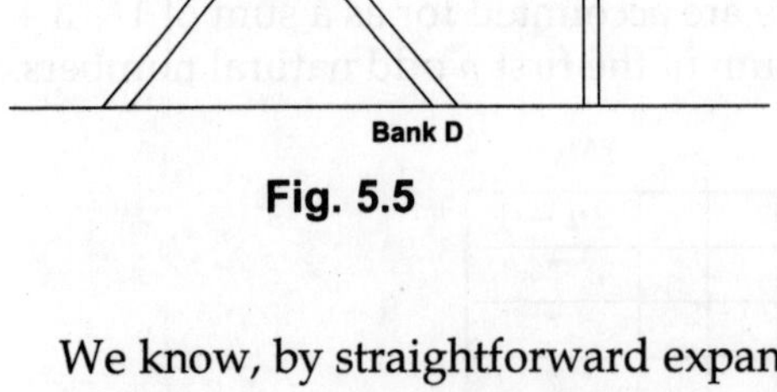

Fig. 5.5

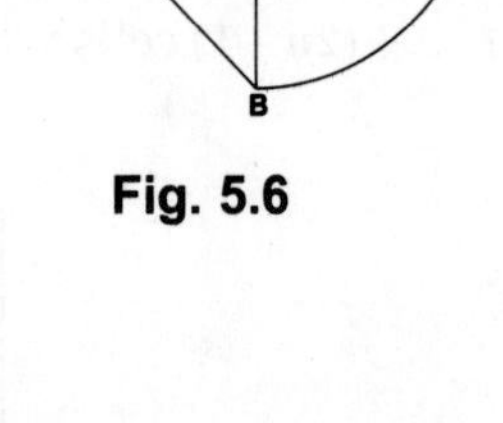

Fig. 5.6

We know, by straightforward expansion, that

$$(a+b)^2 = a^2 + 2ab + b^2, (a+b)^3 = a^3 + 3a^2b + 3ab^2 + b^3.$$

Mathematicians generalised this to any positive integral index, and obtained the following formula for the expansion of $(a+b)^n$:

$$(a+b)^n = \sum_{r=0}^{n} {}^nC_r\, a^r\, b^{n-r}$$

This is called the binomial theorem. It was further generalised to negative and fractional values of the index n.

We know the definition of the inverse of a non-singular matrix, namely matrix B is called the inverse of the non-singular matrix A, if $AB = BA = I$. The definition was generalised and the generalised inverse for any matrix was defined.

We know the Pythagoras theorem states: " The area of the square on the hypotenuse of a right-angled triangle is equal to the sum of the areas of the squares erected on the other two sides of the triangle" or in other words " $c^2 = a^2 + b^2$ " (see Fig. 5.7). A mathematician can generalise this statement (or the problem represented by this statement) in various ways as follows:

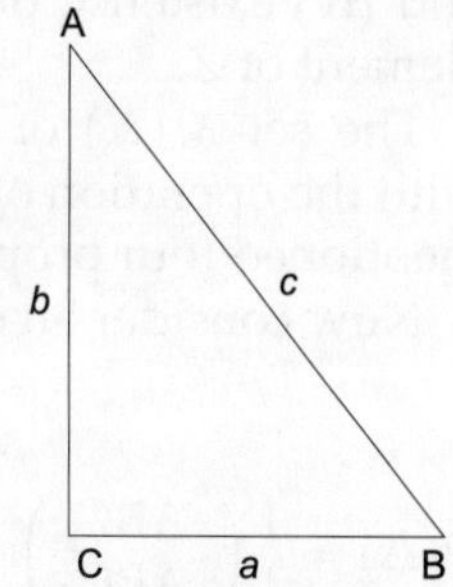

Fig. 5.7

i. What happens if instead of squares, semi-circles or equilateral triangles or any regular figures are erected on the three sides of a right triangle (see diagrams in Fig. 5.8)? It is shown that the area of a regular figure erected on the hypotenuse = sum of the areas of similar regular figures erected on the other two sides of the right triangle.

ii. What happens to the value of c if ∠ C is not a right angle? It is shown that in such a case $c^2 = a^2 + b^2 - 2ab\cos\theta$, where ∠ C = θ. So the Pythagoras theorem becomes a particular case of this general expression for c^2 i.e., when C = 90°.

iii. Instead of 2, if the powers of $a, b, c,$ are equal but an integer ≥ 3, what happens?

It has been shown (see Lecture 8, Section 8.8) that if n is an integer ≥ 3, then no integral values of $a, b, c, (abc \neq 0)$ exist that satisfy the relation $a^n + b^n = c^n$.

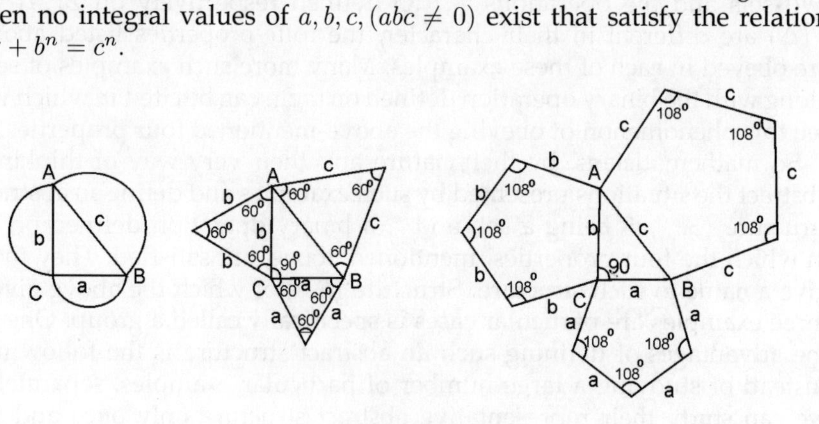

Fig. 5.8

5.20 Abstraction Lies at the Heart of Mathematics

Consider the set $Z = \{\ldots, -3, -2, -1, 0, 1, 2, 3, \ldots\}$ of integers and the usual operation of addition defined on Z. We know that the set Z along with the operation + has the following properties : (i) closure, (ii) associativity of addition, (iii) existence of an identity element (viz., zero), and (iv) existence of inverse (with respect to +) for every non-identity element of Z.

The set $M(N)$ of non-singular matrices of order n (n, finite) along with the operation of multiplication defined on it, also fulfills the above-mentioned four properties.

Now consider an equilateral triangle ABC. Then consider

$$P(\triangle) = \left\{ \begin{pmatrix} \text{ABC} \\ \text{ABC} \end{pmatrix}, \begin{pmatrix} \text{ABC} \\ \text{BCA} \end{pmatrix}, \begin{pmatrix} \text{ABC} \\ \text{BAC} \end{pmatrix}, \begin{pmatrix} \text{ABC} \\ \text{ACB} \end{pmatrix}, \begin{pmatrix} \text{ABC} \\ \text{CAB} \end{pmatrix}, \begin{pmatrix} \text{ABC} \\ \text{CBA} \end{pmatrix} \right\}.$$

Here $\binom{\text{ABC}}{\text{BCA}}$ stands for the position of $\triangle$ABC, if the vertices A, B, C, will shift to the places occupied by the vertices B, C, A before shifting. Similar interpretation will be given to the other members of $P(\triangle)$. Consider the operation, to be denoted by O, on the elements of $P(\triangle)$. The operation can be called "followed by" and is defined as

$$\begin{pmatrix} \text{ABC} \\ \text{BCA} \end{pmatrix} \text{O} \begin{pmatrix} \text{ABC} \\ \text{ACB} \end{pmatrix} = \begin{pmatrix} \text{ABC} \\ \text{CBA} \end{pmatrix}.$$

and similarly for other elements of $P(\triangle)$. Here also we notice that $P(\triangle)$ along with the operation obeys the above-mentioned four properties.

So we see that although the elements of any of the sets $Z, M(N)$, $P(\triangle)$are entirely of different nature than the elements of any of the other two sets and the operations $+, \times$,O defined respectively on $Z, M(N)$, $P(\triangle)$ are different in their character, the four properties listed above are obeyed in each of these examples. Many more such examples of sets along with the binary operation defined on them can be cited in which we see this phenomenon of obeying the above-mentioned four properties.

So mathematicians, by their nature and their very way of thinking, abstract the situations presented by such examples and define an abstract structure $(S,^*)$, S being a set, and *, a binary operation defined on S, in which the four properties, mentioned above, are satisfied. They then give a name to such structure. Structure $(S,^*)$ of which the above given three examples are particular cases is specifically called a group. One of the advantages of defining such an abstract structure is the following. Instead of studying a large number of particular examples, separately, we can study their representative abstract structure only once and all conclusions drawn from such a single study will apply to particular examples. This is very common in mathematics, and mathematicians have come up with many algebraic and topological structures, which occupy a very important part of the study of mathematics. The beauty of such a structure is that we do not know (in fact, need not know for further valid study of structure), concretely the elements of the set and we do not have knowledge about the precise nature of the binary operation. That is why it is, sometimes, jocularly said that "mathematicians do not know what they are talking about". Actually creating and identifying such structures and their study is a strength of mathematics. There are structures in which more than one set and different types of operations on them and among them are defined.

Conclusion

We hope that all of us will remember the various salient features of mathematics, in general, that should form the concerns of our study, and pass them on to others. The references given at the end will shed more light on the above concerns.

Lecture 6

Friendly and Changing Ways of Teaching Mathematics

Abstract

Mathematics is considered by many as one of the greatest and most beautiful creations of the human race. In order to spread its beauty, culture, importance, relevance, and applicability, mathematics must be taught in such a way that everybody becomes an ambassador-at-large of this subject in other fields of human activity. With this in mind certain interesting and student-friendly ways of teaching mathematics are pointed out here. With new developments taking place all around, some changing aspects in teaching this subject have also been brought out.

6.1 Introduction

Everybody knows Lata Mangeshkar, one of the jewels of Indian music. She has established, in the historic city of Pune, a hospital in the memory of her father, Late Deenanath Mangeshkar, a legendary figure in music and dramatics. In one article giving information about this hospital, it was said that the hospital would be patient-friendly. We know how patients are afraid of hospitals and the doctors there. Therefore a hospital becoming patient-friendly is welcome. Indian railways now bring out passenger-friendly time-tables in contrast to their earlier versions. We hear that China is designing an environment-friendly space launch vehicle. Similarly, we hear terms like user-friendly software, investment-friendly economic policies, kids-friendly mobile phones, business-friendly climate, skin-friendly garments, environment-friendly cars etc. It is natural that we would like teaching of any subject in general, and teaching of mathematics in particular, to be student-friendly as the student is the central figure of any teaching activity. If there are no students, there will be no teaching. Teachers, at whatever level, should always try and endeavour to find, discover, and evolve better and better student-friendly ways of teaching our subjects whatever that subject might be. We suggest and mention here some such student-friendly ways for teaching mathematics that we feel will be useful to trigger the imagination of the students and hence make teaching and learning both interesting and appealing. At the same time, we remember the quotation attributed to Einstein, " Make science as simple as possible but no more so ".

6.2 Analogies to Give More Insight in the Subject

Mathematical facts have analogies in other fields [9] of knowledge. This could be exploited for good teaching. We have given two such analogies in Lecture 5, Section 5.7.

V V Karmarkar, sports critic, once quoted: " What cricket do they know who know only cricket? ". This is true of any subject, and in particular, of mathematics. Some knowledge of other fields of study help draw analogies and make study interesting by giving insight. Let us point out proudly that even the Clay Mathematics Institute, Cambridge (Mass., USA) which has offered seven one-million dollar " millennium prizes " for the solutions of seven brain-bending outstandingly difficult problems unveiled by it, has resorted to analogies in order to try to describe some of these problems to novices. This should convince us of the utility and effectiveness of analogies in teaching.

6.3 Use of Stories, Humour, Jokes etc., to Make Teaching Lively

Consider the situation when we teach the theorem which states that the sum of the angles of a triangle is 180°. At this point, we should emphasise to the students that this theorem is from Euclidean plane geometry in which the sides of a triangle are straight-line segments. Tell them further, that our earth being spherical, we cannot draw straight-line segments anywhere on the surface of the earth. Draw students' attention at this stage, to the fact that there exist other geometries known as non-Euclidean geometries that deal with such other situations. Important among these are Riemannian geometry and Bolyai–Labachevsky geometry. In one of these geometries, the sum of the angles of a triangle is greater than 180°, and in the other it is less than 180°. Thus we should bring to the notice of the students that we have three important and equally useful geometries, viz., Euclidean, Riemannian, and Bolyai–Labachevsky. By making the students aware of these geometries, we shall be triggering their thinking as to why the sum of the angles of a triangle is different in these different geometries. They will wonder why mathematics which is considered an exact subject can give different results for the same property of a triangle viz., the sum of its angles. They will be eager to know why this happens. Now we can tell them how Euclid's fifth postulate is the crux of the whole matter. Euclid's plane geometry has five postulates; the fifth one in one of its variant forms (known as the Playfair's axiom) states that from a point outside a given straight line l, one can draw one and only one straight line parallel to l. Euclid himself and many other geometers wanted, if possible, not to regard this as a postulate, but to derive it on the basis of the other four postulates. It was not possible. So geometers turned in the other direction and tried to find the effect of modifying the fifth postulate. Some of them modified the fifth postulate as " one cannot draw a single straight line parallel to a given straight line from a point outside it", while others modified it to say " one can draw any number of straight lines parallel to a given straight line from a point outside it". The two geometries mentioned above arose because of these modifications, and they gave rise to the different theorems, referred to earlier, regarding the sum of the angles of the triangle. All these discussions will emphasis, on the minds of the students, one important aspect of mathematics, namely, that there is nothing like exact or absolute truth in mathematics in which that result lies. In other words, any result or proposition in mathematics has to be consistent with respect to the axioms on which it is based.

To consolidate this important fact of mathematics in the thinking process of students, one can narrate the following humorous story to them. "There were two friends. One was a mathematician, and the other, a politician. They were fast friends throughout even though they belonged to different professions. Once, the politician friend told his mathematician friend: " We are birds of the same feather. We both talk nonsense. The day before yesterday, I came to meet you in your school. You were teaching in a class. I did not want to disturb you; therefore I did not call you outside. But your voice being loud, I could hear what you were teaching. You were telling your students that the sum of the angles of a triangle is 180°. We did study something like this, but I do not remember exactly what it was. So I assumed that what you were telling in the class was correct. I came to meet you yesterday too and you were teaching. But this time I heard you telling your students that the sum of the angles of a triangle is greater then 180°. Now how can this be so? In one class, you tell that the sum is 180°, and in the other you tell that the same sum is greater than 180°. Mathematics being an exact subject, only one of these two statements can and must be true—or am I wrong? We politicians are famed for telling one thing on one platform and exactly the opposite thing on another platform. So I say we both are birds of the same feather; we both talk nonsense ".To this the mathematician replied: "Yes, my dear friend, we both talk nonsense. But there is a difference. I talk consistent nonsense, while you talk inconsistent nonsense. My statements, though they may look contradictory have to be consistent with respect to the axioms with which I started the subject ".

The creativity of a teacher will help him/her construct or devise such relevant and useful stories that will aptly drive a particular topic into the student's mind.

We will tell another story now, that can be told while teaching another facet of mathematics. Students know how to solve the simultaneous equations $x + y = a$, and $x - y = b$, where x and y are the unknowns, and a, b, the known constants. Now suppose you are teaching the students to solve the equations $x + y = c$, and $xy = d$, c and d being known. One way is to derive y as $y = d/x$ from $xy = d$, substitute this y value in $x + y = c$ to get an equation in x alone, solve it to get x, which in turn can be used to get the value of y from one of the earlier equations. Alternatively, to make the situation interesting, one can say that mathematicians are generally lazy, and instead of solving a new problem afresh, they generally try to convert a new problem into a previously known problem (PKP), the method of solving which is known *apriori*. So here the method to solve $x + y = c$, and $xy = d$ by converting it to a PKP is to get $x - y$ from the given equations using $(x - y)^2 = (x + y)^2 - 4xy$. Knowing $x - y$ (say $= g$) thus, one says that you know now how to solve $x + y = c$, and $x - y = g$ as it is a PKP. Mind you, all this is not just for telling a story—it is very common in mathematics to convert a new problem into a PKP, especially in complexity theory in which we decide the complexity of a method of solution of a problem.

To consolidate this fact one can narrate the following very apt humorous story to the students: " A psychologist wanted to study the thinking patterns of different types of scientists. So he brought together at one place, many scientists, each of them belonging to a different field of science—one zoologist, one geologist, one mathematician etc. He arranged an experiment for each of them. The experiment consisted of lifting one specified inanimate object (say a duster for definiteness) from the floor of the room and placing it on a table. The psychologist saw to it that each scientist performed the experiment independently i.e., without observing how it was performed by the other scientists, as he knew that scientists are also known to copy other scientists. There were, of course, many observers to watch the scientists performing the experiment. Each scientist came forward one by one, lifted the duster from the floor, and placed it on the table in the normal way. The mathematician's turn to perform the experiment was at the end. The psychologist and the other observers were eager to see how the mathematician would perform the experiment as mathematicians are generally considered weird and eccentric. The mathematician walked slowly and gracefully, lifted and placed the duster on the table almost exactly the same way as any other scientist did. Here the first part of the experiment was over. The second part of the experiment consisted of lifting the same duster, this time kept on a chair, and placing it on the same table used in the first part of the experiment. Again each scientist came forward, lifted the duster from the chair and placed it on the table in the normal way.

Last came the mathematician; she lifted the duster from the chair, placed it on the floor, pointed her finger from the floor to the table and calmly said that this problem was previously solved (or it was a PKP). This story will obviously cause the class to burst into laughter. We can continue our story like this: "In fact, everybody works this way. An electrical engineer, while building an instrument employing AND gates, NOR gates, OR gates etc., uses only NAND gates in the design map, as every other type of gate can be converted into NAND gates. When I was a student, I stayed in the college hostel. There was a doctor attached to the hostel. Young students studying in colleges are usually quite healthy and rarely need attention from a doctor. My friends in the hostel used to say that our hostel doctor knew only how to cure malaria, and so if a student suffers from dysentery, he would first give medicine that would convert dysentery to malaria, which was a PKP to the doctor. This is just to show that everybody does it, not mathematicians alone".

The mathematical problems, viz., the sum of the angles of a triangle or solving simultaneous equations, taken above, were incidental. A good teacher can find other mathematical situations to befit these stories. A teacher should be able to coin other similar stories for other situations.

Even a small and simple joke can keep the atmosphere of the class lively and help the students understand, appreciate, and digest the related subject matter. Let us take an example. Consider the concept of a "random variable" in probability theory. Actually, a random variable is a function. When one teaches this concept, one can tell the students that naming a new concept is like naming a newly born child. Suppose the name of a girl is Meenakshi; one should not go by the name and think that her eyes would be curved in the shape of a fish. For all we know, she may happen to have round eyes. Similarly, the name of a boy could be Balbhim, but he may not be strong contradicting the feeling one gets by the name Balbhim. So the name of a concept is to be used in the sense given by its definition without attaching any literary meaning to it that might get conveyed by the name. Similar situations exist with many other concepts as well [5].

6.4 Experimentation in Mathematics

Experimentation prepares the students, psychologically, for a new result and serves as a very useful and powerful technique to make the students learn thoroughly with interest and enthusiam. If students learn by their own efforts [7], as they would do during experimentation, they will not have to adopt rote-learning which does not allow insightful thinking.

Experimentation can be profitably employed in high schools before the students are introduced to Euclid's plane geometry in a formal way comprising a sequence of theorems with their proofs. For example, as mentioned in Lecture 5, Section 5.10, students could be asked to draw many different triangles with various shapes and find the sum of the measures of the three angles in the case of each such triangle. In fact, a prize could be announced to those who would be able to draw a triangle, the sum of whose angles is say $200°$ or $150°$. Even after trying for a long time in the class, and at home, the students would find that they cannot get such a triangle and the sum of the angles of any triangle drawn would be $180°$. They could then be told the fact that in Euclid's plane geometry the sum of the measures of all three angles of any triangle is $180°$. They should also be told that they would soon learn to establish this fact, and similar other facts, without resorting to actual measurements, but by arguing it out logically.

Innovative experimentation has another advantage. It makes students realise that there has to be a theoretical way of learning such results without resorting to actual drawings and measurements, as drawings and measurements will involve some inaccuracies. These inaccuracies vary from person to person, and from instrument to instrument, and hence the conclusions based on them cannot be considered to be universally correct—they can only serve as indications of possible correct results which could be taken seriously for theoretical studies. Moreover infinite number of possible types of figures (e.g., triangles in the above mentioned example) exist and we cannot draw all of them before a conclusion or result is announced, as the result is expected to be valid for all possible figures that can be drawn for a given data.

Experimentation can be used with advantage for practically all results that are taught in school mathematics. To cite a few examples, there are results like equality of opposite angles, results about alternate and supplementary angles when a transversal cuts a pair of parallel lines, the result that the sum of the first n odd natural numbers is n^2.

Teachers must experience for themselves the immense joy that students show when they learn through such experimentation. Look also at the great and valuable advantage—results learnt through experimentation are hardly ever forgotten.

6.5 Employing Recreational Mathematics

Recreational mathematics enliven the students interest in learning mathematics. There is always a fear about examination and competition among young ones, even in the minds of brilliant students. So whatever is in the syllabus and taught in the class creates in the student's mind a feeling of dryness and dullness for the subject. First, it is necessary to remove this feeling and make the atmosphere lively. In such an atmosphere, students learn with interest and enthusiasm. We can make use of puzzles, riddles, quizzes, unsolved problems and interesting patterns to create overall liveliness [8]. For this, just as we give homework everyday, we could also give at least one recreational result. The students will be eager to learn about such results. There are plenty of such enlivening mathematics available, like for example, the so-called proof to establish that every triangle is isosceles, and asking them to locate the fallacy in it (see Lecture 5, Section 5.6). Students will be ready to spend any amount of time in trying to understand the facts underlying such results. This will also create in them a desire and interest to learn the regular course material in the syllabus, as these regular matter will be useful in understanding the facts on which the puzzles, riddles, patterns and unsolved problems are based.

To whet the appetite, we shall give two results that will be useful in the strategy of using recreational mathematics advocated here.

We all know what magic squares are. We give here one example of a different kind of magic square. In Fig. 6.1, we have two squares: the one on the left is a magic square with the magic constant 45. This square is related to the one on the right as follows: spell out each entry in the first square, and place the number of letters in the corresponding position in the second square. Thus the first entry is 5, and since the word "five" has 4 letters, the first entry in the second square is 4. Similarly, for the other members in the square. The interesting fact is that the second square so obtained is also a magic square with the magic constant 21. Such magic squares were called alphamagic squares by Lee Sallows. We can get the students interested in finding other alphamagic squares and then ask them to find any property that makes a square an alphamagic square.

5	22	18		Five	Twenty two	Eighteen		4	9	8
28	15	2	→	Twenty eight	Fifteen	Two	→	11	7	3
12	8	25		Twelve	Eight	Twenty five		6	5	10

Fig. 6.1

The second example concerns the interesting property of the number 6174. This was discovered by D R Kaprekar, a high school teacher. Take any four digit number N with at least two unequal digits. One can even take a one, two, or three-digit number and consider it as a four-digit number by padding it with zeros on the left. For example, 1 can be considered as 0001. From the four-digit number chosen, form new numbers A and B by writing the digits of N in decreasing and increasing order, respectively. Find $T(N) = A - B$. T is called the Kaprekar transformation. Kaprekar observed that in at most seven transformations, any four-digit number gets changed to 6174 and the process stops thereafter, since $T(6174) = 7641 - 1467 = 6174$. As an example, note that under $T, 0001 \rightarrow 0999 \rightarrow 8991 \rightarrow 8082 \rightarrow 8532 \rightarrow 6174$.

The number 6174 is appropriately called the "Kaprekar constant". Students can be asked (i) to give a proof of this result and (ii) to find Kaprekar constants in different bases of number systems.

It is appropriate to note here that many interesting problems in recreational mathematics have led to important branches of mathematics. For example, the famous Konigsberg seven bridges problem, (see Lecture 5, Section 5.19) solved by Euler led him to create a useful branch of mathematics viz., graph theory.

6.6 Use of Historical Aspects of Mathematics

The history of mathematics is a great storehouse of information about great problems, fascinating methods of arriving at their solution, and the personalities associated with them. When we trace the progress of the subject, we come across many useful and interesting facts [1, 3]. We realise that an American president, namely James A Garfield had given an independent proof of the Pythagorian theorem. We notice that Mersenne, apart from his contributions to number theory, was famous as a treasurehouse of information for mathematicians. If one wrote to him, asking him something about mathematical problems, either he knew the answer or directed him/her to a possible authority. Reading historical events and facts, we know that even if Fermat is called a "mathematical amateur", it is a great understatement, as his mathematical contributions are tremendous.

Fermat had challenged the then British mathematicians by posing certain problems. These problems came to be known as Fermat's challenge problems. One of them was to find the smallest positive integer x for which $433x^2 + 1$ is a square.

Inspite of the varied great original contributions to mathematics by ancient India, this part of history has not received its due place and recognition by western writers. The actual period in which the mathematicians lived and their discoveries are not correctly acknowledged.

Brahmagupta and Bhaskara II had addressed themselves to Fermat's problems long before they were thought of in the west and had solved them thoroughly. But they do not get a proper place in mathematical history nor are their names attached to the problems and methods of solution in a right way. The French mathematician, Andre Weil, wrote in 1984: "What would have been Fermat's astonishment, if some missionary, just back from India, had told him that his problem had been successfully tackled by native mathematicians almost six centuries earlier!". It is vital that our students should know all this to awaken their national pride. These facts and information will enthuse in them, the spirit of knowledge.

6.7 Changing Ways of Teaching Mathematics

Even educated parents say that they cannot look after their school-children's study of mathematics at home since mathematics taught to their children today is not the same as what they learnt during their student days. Firstly, how can one expect the same mathematics to be taught and that too in the same fashion generation after generation? Subject contents and teaching methodology has to evolve and improve over time. Hence there will be changes in what and how a subject is taught over the years [2, 4, 6]. Secondly, education is not expected to impart just facts and information – it should improve and enhance the capacity of thinking, and the ability to understand on one's own by reading. Hence, if parents are educated in the real sense of the word, they should be able to understand the subject matter by reading books, and if necessary, by discussing with the teachers of their children. By this process, they should be able to help their children, if and when required.

6.8 Changed Methods Due to Impact of Computers

Consider the problem of finding the HCF of two given positive integers. In the days gone by, the method based on finding out actual factors of the integers was taught. Now-a-days, a division-like method has been introduced – the Euclid's algorithm. The method is obviously old, so you may wonder why has this change of method been introduced? For a computer system, finding the quotient and the remainder when one integer is divided by the other is very easy, but finding all the prime factors of a given integer is very hard. Since computers is the "in" thing everywhere, we now teach those methods, in schools and colleges, which are suitable from the computer's point of view. It is not expected that students use computers to find the HCF, but the changed method has found its place in textbooks because of the invention of computers. A new culture has brought changes in methods of teaching.

6.9 Changes Due to Newer Facets of the Subject

Consider the example of evaluating the polynomial, $3x^3 + 4x^2 + 6x + 8$ for $x = 10$. By the usual method of substitution of 10 for x, we will need 6 multiplications, and 3 additions. But if we re-write the above polynomial as $\{(3x+4)x+6\}x+8$, we will be able to evaluate the polynomial in only 3 multiplications, and 3 additions, i.e. in 3 less multiplications. Computers carry out all calculations mainly in terms of additions, subtractions, multiplications, divisions, and comparisons. When we use computers for carrying out huge computations, those methods will be better and preferable which do the work with less number of operations. We should bring in such methods to our textbooks. In the pre-computer era we did not need to find out the number of various operations involved in a method. But now this is a new facet of the subject, useful and necessary because of the advent of computers again. When we teach a method, we should also teach how to analyse that method to find the number of operations needed to solve a problem using that method and compare different methods from this stand-point. This is the change in attitude and approach that is desirable in teaching and writing textbooks in view of the computer revolution that has taken place. This aspect of finding the number of operations required in any method of solving a mathematical problem is very important in the changing ways of teaching mathematics. In fact, this has brought in a new topic – analysis of algorithms – in the fold of mathematics syllabi.

We, without going into details, mention here that even with modern-day sophisticated and fast computers, we cannot solve a big-size or even a moderately big-size real-life problem in a man's life time if the method used to solve it involves $O(n!)$ or $O(e^n)$ steps, n being the size of the problem. A big-size real-life problem can be tackled if a method to solve it exists requiring the total number of operations given by a polynomial in the size of the problem. Therefore we, should also try to discover new methods which require the total number of operations given by a polynomial in the size of the problem. This is exactly what was done by N Karmarkar when he gave a new method to solve a linear programming problem.

6.10 Change Due to Better Proofs

Consider the problem of proving the irrationality of $\sqrt{2}$. Some proofs required that we assume that $\sqrt{2}$, if possible, is expressed in the form p/q in its lowest terms, while some do not. Some proofs are useful to prove irrationality of $\sqrt{2}$ only and cannot be adopted to prove irrationality of $\sqrt{3}$ or $\sqrt{5}$ etc. In our changing ways of teaching mathematics, we should include those methods of proof which can be adopted for similar situations, rather than those which are applicable in particular cases only.

Conclusion

Mathematics is considered by many as a dull and dry subject. The percentages of failures in mathematics at all levels and over the years are generally higher than those in any other subject. Hence, mathematics has always invited attention from all sides – students, parents, teachers, and administrators. There is a saying "once a thief, always a thief" which conveys that once a bad name gets attached to anything or to anybody, its stigma continues perpetually. The same thing has happened with mathematics. It has become the norm to say that mathematics is difficult. To overcome this feeling among many, we have suggested various ways – use of analogies, humorous stories and jokes, experimentation, recreational mathematics, historical aspects – to make mathematics teaching student-friendly.

New discoveries and inventions take place in every human activity. They have an impact on other fields of knowledge; they influence and change the ways of looking at existing problems and procedures. This sometimes gives rise to new subjects or new topics in existing subjects. But it is in the nature of the world that changes – even if these changes are better than existing ways – are resisted, and sometimes opposed inspite of the fact that such opposition is disadvantageous for progress. The only way out of this is to slowly make the resisters appreciate the advantages associated with the changes.

Mathematics is a rigorous subject. We are required to introduce new changes as well as new concepts while teaching it. Initially, we should try to introduce them informally, keeping in mind that these informal ways do not hinder the real understanding of the subject.

Lecture 7

Coping with Reality

Abstract

In this lecture we will illustrate how the mathematics based on Aristotelian logic is inadequate to deal with real-life situations and how fuzzy sets offer better models of reality.

7.1 Introduction

In order to remove paradoxes and in an attempt to keep mathematics free from contradictions, twentieth century mathematicians turned to axiomatisation and formalisation of mathematics. A typical example is the axiomatic set theory whose axioms are presented at the end of Lecture 4.

Axiomatisation together with a formal approach has introduced rigour and precision in mathematics, as never before. But at the same time, as an unavoidable consequence, mathematics has became totally artificial. It has lost its connection with reality. This is fully exhibited in the following quotations.

> As far as laws of mathematics refer to reality, they are not certain. As far as they are certain they do not refer to reality.
>
> **Albert Einstein**

> Introduction of exactness (in mathematics and logic) is artificial and forced... It is not therefore applicable to this terrestrial life but only imaginary celestial existence.
>
> **Bertrand Russell**

> As the complexity of a system increases, our ability to make precise yet significant statements about its behaviour diminishes, until a threshold is reached beyond which precision and significance, (or relevance) become mutually exclusive characters.
>
> **Lotfi Zadeh**

It will be interesting to note that the author of the first quotation was the most renowned physicist, who used mathematics exclusively to establish his theory. The second was a celebrated logician and mathematician. And the third is a meritorious professor of control engineering. All three agree on one issue – at least at some stage, mathematics falls far short of expectations to cope with the real problems of humanity.

7.2 The World of Cognition

In order to get the full import of these quotations let us consider the following three questions:

1. What will be the distance of the planet Neptune from the earth on January, 1, 2020?
2. Who will win maximum gold medals in the 2020 Olympics?
3. Will the world be a better place to live in by 2020?

The first question is precise and it is possible to give a precise answer to it. Sometimes precise answers may not be possible at a certain level of technological development, but there is general consensus that such answers would exist. Questions of this type can be handled with admirably adequate efficiency by present-day mathematics.

The second question falls in a different category. Though the question is precise, a precise answer is not possible till the event actually takes place. These are speculative questions. Though not precise their probabilistic answers can be given with the help of statistical theories.

However, it is the third type of question which is of primary concern to us. Such types of questions cover very vast areas of our cognition. Most real-life problems belong to this category. The formulation of these types of questions is very vague. The meaning may change not only from person to person, but also from time to time for the same person. And yet the question is quite meaningful. All of us will agree that this world needs much to be desired but the prescription for the betterment of the world changes from person to person: Will everybody be happy, if he or she is rich? Let us not labour on happiness. Philosophers have written volumes on the state of happiness and the ways to achieve it. But nobody seems to have benefited from reading those books except their publishers and possibly their authors. What about richness? The word " richness " has many shades, but let us use it in a very mundane earthly sense. How much wealth should one amass, so that one is called rich? Tata is rich. So is Ambani. An average Indian is not rich, so there are some standards on which all of us agree. But such an agreement does not last long. A person whom we consider very rich may be an average middle class commoner in the eyes of Bill Gates. Thus the concept of richness seems to be highly subjective, relative or self-referential. Besides, who should be called rich? One whose annual income is, say, Rs. 5000, 000? And if the answer is affirmative, what about one whose income is a little less than that, say Rs. 4500, 000, annually? And this argument will continue, till a stage is reached where one cannot decide whether a person getting the specified amount should be placed in the category of rich persons or not. For, one may fix any threshold for deciding the richness, but a person bearing little less than that limit need not be considered "non-rich". Thus, the so-called threshold is not only highly arbitrary, but extremely foggy and indiscernible. Yet the question is meaningful. Most questions of the real world are of this nature. They are fuzzy.

7.3 What Causes Fuzziness

There are several factors which contribute to fuzziness. Here we mention some of them.

7.3.1 Natural Language

The first and foremost among the causes of fuzziness is the intrinsic weakness of natural languages. Again it is very much debatable whether it is a strength or a weakness, but there are no two opinions that there is some in-built vagueness in all natural languages. Consider, for example, the following adjectives: A *tall* fellow, an *intelligent* lady, a *handsome* youth,... or for that matter the following sentences; "If you work a *little* harder, then you will get *much* more." "*Heavier* vehicles should be driven *more cautiously*." "The more they change, the more they are the same." Though all these are very meaningful sentences, their meaning is never precise.

7.3.2 Subjective Preferences

Added to the intrinsic fuzziness of a language, there is a subjective element originating from the user. The same word may have different meanings, at different places, to different persons, at different times, and in different circumstances. A young man of twenty-five will consider a fifty-year-old man old. But if you ask the opinion of the fifty-year-old he may reply that he is quite young and energetic. Let us assume that in these types of questions some psychological factors are involved. So let us consider the problem of controlling the " warmness " of water in a shower bath. Here the concept of " warmness " depends on the particular person, at the particular time, of the particular place, in the particular season and above all on the particular mental and physical condition of the user. Note that this problem, unlike the earlier one, is not of academic interest but of economic interest for the manufacturers of the shower-bath equipment and therefore for control engineers.

7.3.3 Inadequacy of Information

Many a time there is no sufficient knowedge of the system. For example, a scientist is always aware that he knows no truth. He may be skeptic even about well-established theories. On the frontiers of knowledge he is always on slippery grounds. If, in addition, the data is inadequate, everything becomes a matter of guesswork and all he has to rely upon is a working hypothesis, based on state-of-the art knowledge and unprovable basic assumptions. These assumptions may be a matter of personal perception, as in a medical or social problem.

Sometimes one has to infer not only from insufficient data but also from information which is not wholly reliable for example, the strength of an enemy in a battle field.

7.3.4 Interdependence of Concepts

The cyclical behaviour of natural phenomena is a favourite concept in ancient Indian philosophy. And a cycle has no cut-point. The seeds of decay, for an Indian philosopher, are present in the growth itself. The transformation of growth into decay is so subtle that you cannot put a demarcation line between them. Let us be more plain. If the demand for a certain commodity increases, its price rises. But the rise in the price results in the decrease of the demand. The end affects the means and the means affects the end. To win elections, a political party has to take some populist measures. However, such measures result in deficit financing and cause inflation and price rise. If the prices rise, it is difficult to contest in the next elections. This interdependence of concepts causes fuzziness in decision making in complex systems like the human body or national economy. Effects of this fuzziness can be easily observed.

7.3.5 Complexity of the System

In many real-life problems, especially where a human element is involved, the system is so complex that it is impossible to control or even to take into account all the affecting factors. Then it becomes a matter of personal choice to decide which factors are to be considered and which are to be ignored. Such a choice in general is not easy.

7.3.6 Cost Effectiveness

Many a time it is theoretically possible to quantify all the parameters of a system. But the cost involved in doing so is so huge, that it is more profitable to ignore certain factors. The choice of relevant factors depends, many times, on personal preferences. This causes fuzziness.

7.4 Paradoxes

Fuzziness of concepts is an open invitation to paradoxes.

7.4.1 Small Heap Paradox

Suppose we have a small heap of stones. Smallness is a fuzzy concept. If we remove a stone from a heap, then of course it will be smaller. But even if we add a stone to the small heap, it will still remain small. Now let us start from the " heap " of a single stone which is definitely small. Since addition of a stone does not affect the smallness of the heap, one can go on adding a stone at a time and still continue to get a " small " heap. This leads to the paradoxical situation where every heap is small.

The bald man's paradox, proposed by Bertrand Russell in 1926, may be described as a dual of the small heap paradox.

7.4.2 Bald Man's Paradox

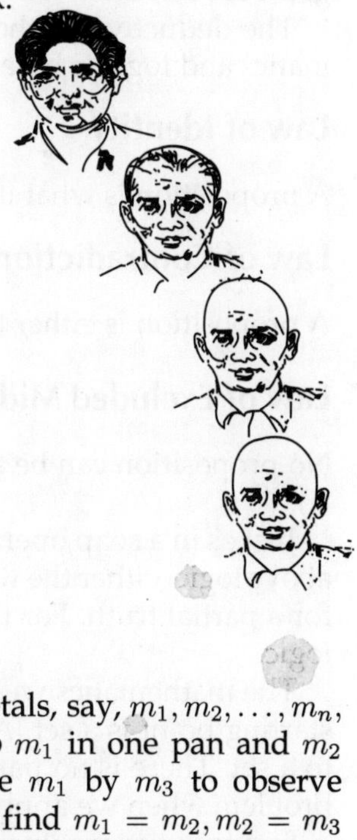

We have a bald man. Can you specify the day from when he would have been declared bald? Of course he was not bald when he was a young man of 25. But thereafter he started losing hair. When he lost his first hair, nobody called him bald, nor after losing the second... and third and .... But today he is called bald so there must have been a hair such that before its fall, he was not bald and after its fall, he was declared bald. Thus the difference between baldness and non-baldness is just one hair!

7.4.3 Poincaré's Paradox

Suppose we are comparing various pieces of metals, say, $m_1, m_2, \ldots, m_n$, in a balance for their relative weight. We keep m_1 in one pan and m_2 in the other to find that $m_1 = m_2$ We replace m_1 by m_3 to observe that $m_2 = m_3$, and continue in this manner to find $m_1 = m_2, m_2 = m_3$ $m_3 = m_4, \ldots, m_{n-1} = m_n$. But at each instance of weighing, there will be a small difference between the two weights, which even the most sensitive machine will fail to detect. And then a stage may come when the machine will show that $m_1 \neq m_n$. This paradox is named after mathematician Poincaré. In describing denseness of real points on an infinite continuum, he observed that adjacent points on the continuum are so indistinguishable from each other that they almost overlap. He describes this situation by the equation $a = b, b = c$, but $a \neq c$.

7.4.4 Epimenides' Paradox

This is an ancient paradox, also known as the paradox of a liar. Epimenides, who himself was a Cretan, says, that all Cretans are liars. Now if Epimenides' statement is true, then being a liar himself, his statement is false. On the other hand, if his statement is false, then he, not being a liar, makes a true statement. Thus the statement is true, if and only if it is false.

7.5 Aristotelian Logic

These paradoxes are the result of our attempt to fit imprecisely expressed concepts into the rigour of the Aristotelian logic. A classic example of putting a square peg in a round hole. Naturally there is an unbridgeable gap between the two.

The deductive method that we employ to derive theorems in mathematics and logic is based on the following three basic Aristotelian laws:

Law of Identity

A proposition is what it is (X is X.)

Law of Contradiction

A proposition is either true or false (X is either Y or not Y.)

Law of Excluded Middle

No proposition can be both, true and false (X cannot be both Y and not Y).

Just as in a soap opera, a character is all good or all bad, we have in the above logic, either the whole truth or the whole untruth. There is no room for a partial truth. For this reason Aristotelian logic is called two-valued logic.

The mathematics we study is based on the two-valued logic. Here the starting point is a set. An object can either belong to a set or not belong to a set. There is no partial belonging to the set. This situation creates a problem when we apply set theory to a real-life situation.

Suppose we are interested in finding the set of poor people in India. According to the government notification, any citizen of India whose yearly earning is Rs. 25000/- or less is considered economically backward (an euphemism for poor). Let U denote the set of citizens of India and let $E(x)$ stand for "yearly income of Mr. x". Thus the set P of poor people, according to this definition is $P = \{x \in U | E(x) \leq 25000\}$. Suppose Raam earns Rs 25000/- per annum and his brother Laxman, Rs 25001/- p.a. Clearly, mathematically and also according to the goverment rule, Raam belongs to P, while Laxman does not. But this is not recreational mathematics or a classroom exercise.

Raam is going to receive cash benefits. His son and daughter are going to get free education. His family is going to get food at a concessional rate. Possibly, he may even get a small residential accommodation, freely. All this will be denied to Laxman because he is richer than his brother by a rupee, annually! This is ridiculous.

The usual remedy to this problem is to " condone " one rupee. In plain terms it means if earnings of x and y differ by 1 rupee, we treat both of them as poor (i.e., they are in P) or as non-poor (i.e., they are not in P) since their financial status is regarded as the same. We denote the financial status of Mr. x by symbol $S(x)$. Clearly S(Raam)= S(Laxman).

Suppose a friend of Laxman, namely Krishna earns Rs 25002/- p.a. By our definition Laxman, and Krishna have the same status, i.e., S(Laxman)= S(Krishna). But Raam and Krishna do not have the same financial status for their income differs by Rs 2/-. In other words

$$S(\text{Raam}) = S(\text{Laxman});$$

$$S(\text{Laxman}) = S(\text{Krishna}) \text{ but } S(\text{Raam}) \neq S(\text{Krishna}).$$

Thus condoning one rupee (and for that matter any number of rupees) lands us in Poincaré's paradox.

To overcome this difficulty suppose we obtain a Government decree that if $S(x) = S(y)$ and $S(y) = S(z)$, then we assume that $S(x) = S(z)$. But a moment's scrutiny shows that the decree does not solve the problem.

Suppose we arrange elements of U as $x_0, x_1, x_2, \ldots, x_n$ in such a way that the earning of x_ϕ is 0, that of x_1 is Rs.1/- per year,..., that of x_n is Rs. n per year. It follows that as earnings of two citizens in succession differ only by a rupee, we have $S(x_0) = S(x_1), S(x_1) = S(x_2), S(x_1), \ldots, S(x_{n-1}) = S(x_n)$. And then by the Government decree, $S(x_0) = S(x_1) = \ldots = S(x_n)$, that is, the financial status of all citizens $S(x_0) = S(x_1) = \ldots S(x_n)$ is the same. This is like the small heap paradox, mentioned earlier which makes a mockery of the concept of defining poverty.

Einstein's quotation given at the beginning should be understood in the light of this fact.

7.6 Fuzzy Set: Compromise with Reality

Professor Lotfi Zadeh suggests a way out of this imbroglio by defining a fussy set. He does not answer all the questions, but he does make things easier for us. Moreover, in the process, he does not disturb the already developed mathematics.

He observes that though a line of demarcation, like Rs 25000/- in the above example, does not satisfactorily define P, there is no controversy over the status of X_{25000} as poor and of X_{100000} as non-poor. Therefore, while moving from X_{25000} to X_{100000}, some change does take place. The change is not abrupt. It is gradual. Therefore, there may not be sharp dividing lines between the poor and others, but a grey area, some " no-man's land " which lies between them. How small or how large that grey area is, depends on the fuzziness of the concept. The sharp dividing line may be well-represented by assigning value 0 to those elements of U which do not belong to P and the value 1 to those which belong to P. The grey area will be represented by assigning values between 0 and 1. Thus in the present example $X_0, X_1, \ldots, X_{25000}$ may be assigned the value 1 and $X_{1000000}$, onwards may be assigned the value 0, X_{500000} may have value 0.5, while X_{300000} may have the value 0.30 attached to it. Thus Zadeh attaches a unique grade to each element of U, to be a member of P. This rule of defining grade membership of a set is called a fuzzy set.

More generally, if A is a fuzzy concept, meaningful for every element x of the universal set U and the grade of x to be a member of A, is denoted by $A(x)$, then $A(x)$ is a real number lying between 0 and 1. The equation $A(x) = 0$ stands for the statement, " x is not a member of A "; $A(x) = 0.5$ for the statement " x may or may not be a member of A "; $A(x) = 0.99$ for, " it is almost surely a member of A ", $A(x) = 0.001$ for, " It is almost impossible for X to be a member of A ", ... etc. In this way Zadeh converts a " *linguistic variable" into a " numerical variable.* " The rule of assigning to each x of U, a unique value $A(x)$ in the set of all real numbers between 0 and 1, (including both 0 and 1) is called a fuzzy set A.

The logician Max Black has described three types of inexactness.

a. **Generality:** A word in the description encompasses much more than intended by a speaker.

b. **Ambiguity:** A word used by the speaker stands for more than one distinguishable concept.

c. **Vagueness:** The word does not have sharply defined jurisdiction.

The definition of a fuzzy set given above takes care of all the three types of inexactness. The generality can be taken care of by choosing the universal set U large enough. The ambiguity can be accommodated by giving different members of U, approximately the same grade of membership. The vagueness is managed by attaching, if necessary, the whole range of values between 0 and 1.

The classical theory of sets resolved the long-standing paradoxes of Zeno (Lectures 2 and 3). The axiomatic set theory avoids paradoxes such as those of Russell's and Berry's. The fuzzy set theory resolves the paradoxes mentioned in Section 7.4.

7.7 Resolution of Paradoxes

In the fuzzy set theory, the small heap paradox disappears, if we give decreasing membership-grade to smallness, as the stones are added to the heap. Poincaré's paradox similarly disappears by suitably defining the grade membership function from the set of pairs of real numbers into the set $[0, 1]$. Epimenides' paradox is resolved by assigning value 0.5 to his statement.

7.8 Fuzzy Sets and Probability Theory

The theory of probability, like fuzzy sets, deals with uncertainty. Both tackle the problem of uncertainty by considering functions whose values lie between 0 and 1. But the uncertainty in probability theory is objective, while that of the fuzzy set theory is subjective. To be more explicit, consider the example of tossing a coin. The probability of getting a head is 1/2, *provided* the coin is unbiased. But how do we decide that the coin is unbiased? There is a positive probability that all the outcomes are the same even if the coin is unbiased! The situation will not change even if we toss the coin a thousand times or any number of times. Thus the uncertainty related to the unbiasedness of the coin is fuzzy, while that of the outcome – once the first issue is settled – is probabilistic.

The concept of a fuzzy set goes a step ahead of probability in the sense that a fuzzy set can assume values in any bounded lattice and not necessarily in the interval $[0, 1]$.

7.9 Multi-valued Logic and Fuzzy Sets

The basic concept in the fuzzy set theory that "every thing is a matter of degree" dates back to the first quarter of the twentieth century. In the 1920s, the Polish logician Jan Lukasiewicz put forward the principle of multi-valued truth values between 0 and 1. In fuzzy sets we consider all the values between 0 and 1 (if necessary). In 1937, the logician, philosopher Max Black applied multi-valued logic to lists. Lists are some sets of objects. Black called them "vague". In 1965, almost thirty years after Black and forty-five years after Lukasiewicz, Zadeh applied the logic to every object in a set and produced a complete algebra of fuzzy sets.

The multi-valued logic did not go far. It stopped at two quantifiers – "all" and "some" But fuzzy logic can have any number of quantifiers like "few", "most", "very few", "almost all", "several", "quite a few" – in principle an infinity of quantifiers. Besides, in fuzzy logic, a truth itself can be fuzzy.

However the concept of a fuzzy set was initiated by a technologist and not a philosopher. Therefore, its strength lies in its applicability to real-life situations.

7.10 Applications of Fuzzy Sets

The mathematics based on two-valued logic has been remarkably successful in solving problems in physical sciences and technology, where systems have been relatively less complicated and the problems have been more exactly defined. Considering the simplicity of mathematical tools, their achievements are amazing. But since fuzzy logic is much better suited to describe the real world, which is intrinsically fuzzy, the mathematics based on fuzzy sets becomes a more powerful tool to solve real-life problems. This explains the ever-increasing use of fuzzy sets in social sciences, psychology, linguistics, medicines, communication systems, informatics, neural network, pattern recognition, robotics, and many other fields, where knowledge is incomplete, information is imprecise or ideas vague.

However, since early fuzzy theorists have been control engineers, it is quite natural that the early uses of fuzzy systems was in control theories. Here we mention some of the more widely known applications.

1. In the mid-1970s, Ebrahim H Mamdani of the Imperial College of Science, Technology and Medicine, London, designed the first fuzzy control for a steam engine.

2. In 1980, a contracting firm F L Smidth & Co. of Copenhagen, used fuzzy systems to oversee its construction operations.

3. In 1985, Bell Laboratory built the first digital fuzzy chip. It processed 16 simple rules in 12.5 microseconds at the rate of 0.08 million fuzzy logical inferences per second.

4. The most famous application of fuzzy systems, of course, is the subway car control, used in Sendai, Japan. This is a complete engineering system and not a prototype or an experimental one. It has been in commercial use since 1987. Professor Seiji Yasunobu of the Institute of Engineering Mechanics, University of Tsubuka, Japan, has designed the system. It operates through 17 stations, over 15 km. By Tokyo or Osaka standards, Sendai is not a huge system. Still it serves 1000,000 people daily. There has been no accident since the time the system has been installed. The new system has also resulted in a 10% reduction in energy consumption.

The Sendai subway demonstrates that it is possible to use experts' knowledge to design control laws and fuzzy theory as a means to translate natural language information into a control strategy.

5. One of the most complex fuzzy systems is a model of a helicopter, designed by Professor Michio Sugeno of the Tokyo Institute of Technology. The helicopter responds to 13 oral commands like " up ", " down ", and " hover ". The fuzzy control can make the craft hover in a terrain difficult for a human pilot.
6. Omran Corporation, an Iraqi–Japanese syndicate, oversees five medical databases in health management systems for big firms. It uses fuzzy systems with 500 rules and gives personalised medical service to 10, 000 people.
7. Hitachi and Yamaichi securities are using fuzzy rules to take decisions in the stock market.
8. In Germany a special programme system called FUZSIM has been developed for simulating a static and dynamic complex system using a fuzzy model. Based on this system, a model for water flow and water level for the river Elbe was developed and forecasts were made. The fuzzy model appeared to be more suitable as the accuracy of data was not assured.
9. In Czechoslovakia, a system called CONFUCIUS was developed to realise approximate reasoning. It works with 30 variables and can describe a model with several hundred conditional statements. About 100 problems are reported to have been solved by using this system.

The list can be lengthened considerably. Japan has marketed many consumer products like washing machines, refrigerators, vacuum cleaners, micro-wave ovens, braking systems, fuel injectors and many others using fuzzy technologies. In fact, it is out of fashion in Japan to use a gadget which does not apply fuzzy logic. According to its Ministry of International Trade and Industry, Japan has produced fuzzy products worth $ 2000,000.000.

7.11 Limitations of the Fuzzy Theory

The first paper on the fuzzy set appeared in the year 1965. By the year 1970, there were 25 papers. The number reached 227 during the next five years. In the beginning of 1994, the number of papers published on fuzzy theory and its applications reached the colossal figure of 15,000. The first journal devoted exclusively to fuzzy sets and systems started publication in the year 1978. At present there are many international journals which publish papers exclusively on fuzzy theory and technology. In addition many journals devoted to mathematics and engineering disciplines, publish papers on the subject. The International Fuzzy Systems Association, the first worldwide organisation dedicated to the support and development of the theory of fuzzy sets and technology was established in 1984. Now there are many societies all over the world working towards the same goal.

However, even the founding father of the fuzzy set theory does not claim that it will give ultimate answers to all the problems posed in the real world. The weakest point in the system is the need to determine a fuzzy rule. At present the fuzzy consumer products in the market rely on the rules supplied by experts. This is far from ideal. Fuzzy sets are introduced to mathematise subjective ambiguity. As such, a genuine fuzzy system product should cater to the needs of each consumer.

At present most fuzzy systems have been control systems with few variables. If we want to model an economy, we would need a very large number of variables. The fuzziness in natural language is probably the most formidable obstacle. Constructing a computer which will obey oral commands is a distant dream. In such a scenario there may be no experts to rely upon. Commonsense may be useless and neural nets set up to learn the rules for a model may have no data to work with.

Control systems work on electronic gadgets, which are essentially two-state devices. At present, attempts are being made to compensate for this deficiency of computer hardware by suitable modifications in the software. The human brain has a capacity to discard inessential information and concentrate on whatever is relevant. An electronic machine will require a lot of time to perform such an act. Thus using a two-valued device to solve fuzzy-valued problems is not an efficient way of getting the work done. Let us hope that the problem will be overcome some day by the construction of a non-electronic computer, may be a chemical or molecular one, which works along the lines of the human brain.

What is said of a computer holds good for the fuzzy set theory itself. Even though we express fuzzy logic through fuzzy sets, we are not completely out of the set theory based on two-valued logic. A fuzzy set being a well-defined function, is not a fuzzy concept. This is clearly a handicap. It does not allow a fuzzy set to grasp the essence of vagueness. Attempts are being made to give a categorical foundation to fuzzy sets and thus avoid the impasse.

There are some other attempts to cope with the uncertainty in real-life situations. In 1975, a group of mathematicians lead by P Vopenka proposed the concept of " alternative set theory. " This approach is more radical than the fuzzy sets in the sense that it does not refer to the classical set theory. The concept of a semi-set in the alternative set theory and the vagueness of an object, both being equally imaginary, a semi-set is better qualified to catch the evasive spirit of vagueness. A fuzzy set can be a reasonable approximation of a semi-set.

The concept of rough sets is another approach to describe indiscernibility. It was introduced by Z Pawlak of the Institute of Computer Science, Warsaw University of Technology. It considers finite sets and equivalence relations on them. Finite sets are sufficient from the point of view of a user. But indiscernibility is one aspect of vagueness. The vagueness of natural languages cannot be captured by a rough set. Probably it may be more rewarding to use it in conjunction with fuzzy sets. Some attempts have already been made in this direction.

Conclusion

The fuzzy set theory is yet to find a place in mainstream mathematics. It has not solved any existing problems in mathematics. But in mathematics, any generalisation takes a long time to gain acceptance. These are issues which only time can settle. At present we can say with confidence that the concept of fuzzy sets does generalise many existing concepts in mathematics. And generalisation is an aim of mathematics. Moreover, how can anyone ignore a tool which is as useful as fuzzy sets?

Arresting the imprecision of reality within the rigid framework of mathematics may be a dream. But only the human brain is blessed with the capacity to dream. And the progress of science is shaped by such dreams. Students can frame many projects after reading references [1] to [9].

Lecture 8

Conjectures in Mathematics

Abstract

Mathematics is often compared with a game which is not only to be observed but also one in which one must participate wholeheartedly. When we participate, we gain certain insights, observe certain patterns and notice some characteristic properties of the situation represented by that game. From these patterns and/or properties, one tends to make certain intelligent surmises or guesses. We are not able to immediately come up with proofs, about the validity of those surmises as compulsorily required in mathematics. But at the same time, one does develop strong beliefs about the truth of these guesses—enough to declare them as conjectures. In time, these conjectures are proved or disproved. We present here some such conjectures and some noteworthy information about them.

8.1 Introduction

A conjecture in mathematics is an intuitive and shrewd guess made by a person with good mathematical insight. Throughout the history of mathematics, conjectures have been made by many research workers. Some of them have been proved and some disproved at some later date. It is a great day for mathematics when a certain conjecture is proved or disproved. The longer the time gap between the day a conjecture is proposed and the day on which it is proved or disproved, the better, in general, is the quality and the strength of the conjecture. There is no point in making a conjecture, guess or surmise which would be found correct or would be demolished within a few hours, days or so. There are certain conjectures in mathematics which have remained unsettled, this way or that, for centuries.

One of the most famous and difficult conjectures in mathematics is the one known as the Riemann hypothesis. It has not been proved till today. Its importance and fascination can be understood by the fact that the renowned German mathematician, David Hilbert, once said that, were he awakened after having slept for a thousand years, his first question would be, has the Riemann hypothesis been proved?

8.2 Graeco-Latin Squares

The first conjecture we shall take up for discussion will be introduced through a story. Consider the sixteen picture cards from the usual pack of playing cards. They are the 4 aces, 4 kings, 4 queens and 4 jacks. These 16 cards can be classified in two different ways: (i) according to their denominations, viz., ace, king, queen, jack, and (ii) according to their suit, viz., club, diamond, heart, spade. Now suppose that we want to arrange these 16 picture cards in a 4 × 4 square (i.e., a square having 4 rows and 4 columns) in such a way that every denomination and every suit must occur once and only once in each row and in each column. Now, we know that when a mathematician wants to solve this problem, he/she will not generally use the actual playing cards; instead he/she will use symbols to indicate the denominations and suits. Let the Latin (or Roman) letters A, B, C, D stand for the denominations namely ace, king, queen, jack respectively and let the Greek letters α, β, χ, δ denote the four suits namely club, diamond, heart and spade respectively. Thus Aα indicates the club ace, and similarly $A\beta$, $B\alpha$ etc. Thus we have the 16 picture cards represented by Aβ, Aχ, Aδ, Bβ,. . ., Dδ,. Figure 8.1 then gives one of the arrangements that satisfies the requirements laid down above by us. Observe that each Latin and each Greek letter occurs once and only once in each row and each column of the 4 × 4 square. Also observe that all the 16 possible representations or combinations Aα, . . .,Dδ have found places in the cells of the square.

Aα	Bβ	Cχ	Dδ
Bβ	Aδ	Dα	Cβ
Cδ	Dχ	Aβ	Bα
Dβ	Cα	Bδ	Aχ

Fig. 8.1

A	B	C	D
B	A	D	C
C	D	A	B
D	C	B	A

α	β	χ	δ
χ	δ	α	β
δ	χ	β	α
β	α	δ	χ

Fig. 8.2

Such a square configuration is called a Graeco-Latin square of order 4. The name is so given because the Greek and Latin letters are used in its construction. If some of our ancestors would have discovered it first, it would have, perhaps been named as Kannada-Tamil square or Devanagari-Telugu square or the like. We have lost that opportunity, I think.

One can see that a Graeco-Latin square of order 4, given in Fig. 8.1 can be obtained by super-imposing on each other the two squares given in Fig. 8.2. In each of the squares of Fig. 8.2, four different symbols are used; in one, symbols used are A, B, C, D, while in the other they are $\alpha, \beta, \chi, \delta$. Actual symbols used are immaterial; one could use, for example, $1, 2, 3, 4$ if one likes. What is important however, is that each symbol used must occur once and only once in each row and in each column of the square. One can verify that this is so in the case of each of the squares of Fig. 8.2. A square satisfying this property is called a Latin square irrespective of the nature of the symbols used in constructing the square (maybe, the first time such a square was constructed, Latin letters were used). Thus each of the two squares in Fig. 8.2 is a Latin square.

Two Latin squares, which when super-imposed gives a Graeco-Latin square, are called orthogonal Latin squares. The two Latin squares of Fig. 8.2 are thus orthogonal Latin squares (orthogonal to each other). One can also notice that the second Latin square of Fig 8.2 is obtainable from the first by establishing a one-one correspondence between the Latin and Greek letters used in them and by suitably re-arranging the rows of the first square. If we want to construct all possible Graeco-Latin squares by first systematically enumerating all possible Latin squares and super-imposing two using every possible pair out of them, and verifying whether what we get is a Graeco-Latin square or not, we should first try the exercise with Latin squares of order 3. This will give us the feeling, idea, and insight of the amount of effort involved in the construction of Latin and Graeco-Latin squares of higher orders. We can prove that there are at least $[n!(n-1)!(n-2)!\ldots 2!1!]$ Latin squares of order n. Now we can verify that there are only 12 Latin squares of order 3. The number of possible Latin squares increases rapidly as n increases. There are 576 Latin squares of order 4, and 161280 of order 5. Further, there are never more than $n-1$ mutually orthogonal Latin squares of order n.

We know that a mathematician is never satisfied by solving only a particular specific problem; he/she is always interested in generalising it. So the question now is: can we have a Graeco-Latin square of order n for any positive integer n? The famous mathematician Euler (1707–1783) tackled this problem. He could not prove his result, but on the basis of his studies, he arrived at a considered opinion which he presented as a conjecture: " A Graeco-Latin square of an evenly even order does not exist (i.e., cannot be constructed by anybody) ". A positive integer is evenly even if it is of the form $4n+2$, when $n = 0, 1, 2, \ldots$ Thus, according to Euler's conjecture, Graeco-Latin squares of order $2, 6, 10, \ldots$ do not exist and hence nobody can construct them. One can easily verify, by trying out all possibilities (which is known as the method of complete enumeration or the method of exhaustive verification), that a Graeco-Latin square of order 2 cannot exist. In the case of order 6, French mathematician G Tarry, in 1901, using mechanical aids, verified that Graeco-Latin squares of order 6 do not exist.

At this stage we will narrate another relevant story. One day, a Czar ordered his commander-in-chief to collect 36 officers from his army, belonging to 6 different ranks (like captain, major etc.) and to 6 different regiments (like our Rajputana regiment) taking exactly one officer of each of the ranks, from each of the regiments, and make them stand in a 6×6 square so that in each row and in each column there stands one and only one person belonging to each rank and each regiment. The C-in-C could not achieve this task and you can imagine what happened to him in the regime of the Czar. After reading about Euler's conjecture, one can understand why the C-in-C could not accomplish the task assigned to him—he was asked, in fact, to construct a 6×6 Graeco-Latin square and there is no way it can exist, as stated above.

Now, how about a Graeco-Latin square of order 10, and higher evenly even order? Even for the fastest computer of the world, it was almost impossible to completely enumerate all possible cases and verify Euler's propositions for Latin squares of even order 10. So mathematics (and not the mere computation of the complete enumeration variety) was the only hope to resolve the issue posed by Euler.

The D-day came when Euler's conjecture was disproved. Two Indian mathematicians were associated with this event—R C Bose and S S Shrikhande. They proved that a Graeco-Latin square of order 6 does not exist (as predicted by Euler and verified by Tarry), but it can be constructed for any other order $4n + 2, (n \geq 2)$. They, in fact, also gave a concrete example of a Graeco-Latin square of order 10. These mathematicians came to be known as "Euler's Spoilers" by their friends, as they spoiled (so to say) Euler's conjecture.

An example of a 10×10 Graeco-Latin square is given in Fig. 8.3. Here digits have been used instead of Greek and Roman letters. From this, we can separately obtain two 10×10 squares, one formed by keeping only the first digit from each of the cells in it, and the second obtained by retaining only the second digit of each of the cells. These two squares will be (orthogonal) Latin squares in their own right. Their super-imposition has given us the above Graeco-Latin square.

We notice that the 3×3 square at the right-hand bottom corner of the two new 10×10 Graeco-Latin squares is itself a Graeco-Latin square. Bose, Shrikhande (along with Parker this time), constructed many different Graeco-Latin squares of order 10, and each of them contained such a Graeco-Latin square of order 3.

00	47	18	76	29	93	85	34	61	52
86	11	57	28	70	39	94	45	02	63
95	80	22	67	38	71	49	56	13	04
59	96	81	33	07	48	72	60	24	15
73	69	90	82	44	17	58	01	35	26
68	74	09	91	83	55	27	12	46	30
37	08	75	19	92	84	66	23	50	41
14	25	36	40	51	62	03	77	88	99
21	32	43	54	65	06	10	89	97	78
42	53	64	05	16	20	31	98	79	87

Fig. 8.3

The disproof of Euler's conjecture was announced at the annual meeting of the American Mathematical Society in April 1959. The proof of a conjecture in advanced group theory was also announced at that meeting. Thus the meeting was a mathematical event of the first magnitude.

One may wonder and ask: " What is the use of Graeco-Latin squares in practice apart from the fun derived in creating certain configurations and patterns using certain symbols? ". Actually they are extremely useful for applications in designing experiments in biology, agriculture, medicine, sociology, marketing etc. Let us explain with an example. Suppose a medical researcher wants to examine the effects of 7 different types of injections on persons coming from 7 different age brackets, 7 different weight groups and 7 different stages of the same disease. Then the most efficient layout for the researcher's experiment will be given by a 7×7 Graeco-Latin square selected randomly from all possible squares of that order. Its 7 rows will represent 7 different age brackets; its 7 columns will represent 7 different weight groups; the 7 different Latin symbols will represent 7 different stages of the disease in patients , and the 7 different Greek symbols will represent 7 different types of injections. Thus the researcher can conduct his experiment with only 49 patients instead of the $7 \times 7 \times 7 \times 7$ patients that would be normally considered necessary. When a Graeco-Latin square design is used, its rows take care of one variable (like age bracket in the above example), columns take care of another (like weight group), the Latin symbols, the third variable (like stage of the disease in a patient), and the Greek symbols, the fourth (like type of injection). It thus takes into consideration 4 different sources of variation that contribute to or affect the observations.

We discussed the conjecture related to Graeco-Latin squares first because two Indian mathematicians of recent time were associated with resolving the conjecture [3]. Many a time, students and teachers ask: Have there been any renowned mathematicians produced in India after Ramanujan. Harish-Chandra, R C Bose, C R Rao, and Shreeram Abhyankar are some of the most outstanding renowned mathematicians of India, coming after Ramanujan. Incidentally, they have all come from different parts of India and in some way this shows that it is not the soil of a particular part of India that is more conducive for mathematicians to be born. What is really needed is proper and unbiased spotting, nurturing and encouraging of budding mathematicians. Let us hope that the teachers of mathematics do their duty with due devotion and dedication in this respect.

8.3 Euler's Number Theory Conjecture

Euler is renowned for being associated with many easy-to-state-and-understand but difficult-to-tackle propositions like the Graeco-Latin square conjecture discussed in Section 8.2. We now take up another conjecture by Euler, resolved as late as in 1988.

Euler had conjectured that there exist no integers a, b, c, d such that $a^4+b^4+c^4 = d^4$. Fortunately or unfortunately (we cannot say which), this conjecture of Euler was also disproved when Noam D Elkies of Harvard University (USA) found in 1988 that $a = 2682440, b = 15365639, c = 18796760$ and $d = 20615673$ satisfy the relation $a^4 + b^4 + c^4 = d^4$. This coming up with a counter-example by Elkies and providing a disproof of Euler's conjecture involves some good mathematics and not just a computer search. Again, Roger Frye of Thinking Machine Corporation at Cambridge (Massachussetts, USA) gave another example, viz., $a = 95800, b = 217519, c = 414560$ and $d = 422481$, with which also we get $a^4 + b^4 + c^4 = d^4$. We notice that Frye's a, b, c, d, are smaller than those of Elkies. Frye got his a, b, c, d using 110 hours of computer time. Now it is known that there exist infinitely many quadruples a, b, c, d satisfying $a^4 + b^4 + c^4 = d^4$, but they are sparsely distributed.

In fact, Euler's conjecture in the above paragraph is a particular case $(n = 4)$ of the general conjecture: "For every positive integer n, it is possible for n nth powers to add to an nth power (a famous manifestation of this for $n = 2$ being the Pythagoras theorem), but not for $n - 1$ to dc so". In 1966 L J Lender and T R Parkin found the first counter-example to this: $27^5 + 84^5 + 110^5 + 135^5 = 144^5$. This remained the only example till 1988 when Elkies gave the counter-example stated above.

8.4 Kaprekar's Conjecture

Dattatreya Ramachandra Kaprekar (1905–1986) [6,7,8] was a high school teacher at Deolali (Maharashtra, India), who descovered many interesting properties in recreational number theory. We explain below the conjecture stated by Kaprekar.

Consider the prime 31. Add its digits to the number itself. We get $31 + 3 + 1 = 35$ which is a composite. Thus we get a composite number from a prime in just one step – adding all the individual digits of the prime to itself. Some more primes of this type are 17, 41, 109, 3001 and 2003. Now consider the prime 127. Add to it all its digits to get $127 + 1 + 2 + 7 = 137$ which is also a prime. Do the same thing to it to get $137 + 1 + 3 + 7 = 148$ which is a composite number. Here we get a composite number, starting from a prime, in two steps. Some other examples of primes of this type are 307, 587, 1009, 1061 and 1087. So our procedure is to take a prime, add all its individual digits to get a new number, repeat the same procedure on it if it is a prime and continue doing this till one gets a composite number. Some examples of primes for which we need three steps to arrive at a composite number are 11, 101, 149, 167, 367, 479 and 1409. Some examples of primes for which we need four steps to reach a composite number are 277 and 1559. Kaprekar's conjecture is that there exists no prime for which we need more than four steps to get a composite number by the above-described procedure.

Kaprekar's conjecture was disproved as recently as in November 2001 by a Physics B Sc. final-year student, Mr. Vishal H. Joshi, from Jamnagar (Gujarat, India). He produced many primes which require 5 or 6 steps to reach a composite number. To disprove a conjecture, one just needs one counter-example. From Vishal Joshi's collection, we shall give four examples – two requiring 5 steps and two, six steps. They are (i) prime number 37783 which becomes successively $37783+28 = 37811$, $37811+20 = 37831$, $37831 + 22 = 37853$, $37853 + 26 = 37879$, $37879 + 34 = 37913$. Till the fourth step we get primes; at the 5th step, we get a composite number 37913 whose factors are 31 and 1223. (ii) Prime number 85601 at the end of the 5th step becomes composite $85726 = 2 \times 42863$. All the previous 4 steps produced primes: $85601 \to 85621 \to 85643 \to 85669 \to 85703$; the last one finally yields the composite 85726. (iii) Prime number 516493 yields primes (viz. 516521, 516541, 516563, 516589, 516623) in the first five consecutive steps, and the sixth step produces the composite $516646 = 2 \times 13 \times 31 \times 641$. (iv) When the required procedure of digits addition is applied to the prime 1885943, we successively get 1885981, 1886021, 1886047, 1886081, 1886113 which are primes. Then the 6th step gives the composite $1886141 = 12491 \times 151$.

8.5 Catalan's Conjecture

This is a very simple looking conjecture thought up by E C Catalan. It states that the only two consecutive positive integers which are perfect powers are 8 and 9. It was not proved till 2003 when P Mihailescu published his proof in *J.Reine Angeus. Math* (*Crelle's Journal*) 572(2004): 167–195 [9].

8.6 Bertrand's Postulate (Now a Theorem)

The statement "*For every x greater than 1, there exists a prime p such that $x < p < 2x$*" is known as Bertrand's postulate. Bertrand stated it in 1845. Pafnuty Lvovich Tchebysheff, the Russian mathematician proved it in 1852. Tchebysheff's proof was very complicated. Later Ramanujan and Paul Erdös (at the age of 17) (1913–1996) gave different alternative proofs. This theorem is immediately handy in proving that primes are infinite in number. So Bertrand's postulate which was a conjecture during 1845–1852, is now a theorem.

One surprising consequence of this theorem is that there are at least three primes having exactly n digits, where n is any positive integer.

Bertrand's postulate is important as can be seen by the fact that it has been proved by three different renowned mathematicians separately. But surprisingly it is yet not known whether a prime lies between the square of any number greater than 1 and the square of its consecutive number i.e., for every $x > 1$, there exists a prime p such that $x^2 < p < (x+1)^2$.

8.7 Four Colour Conjecture (Now a Theorem)

The four colour conjecture states that four colours are sufficient to colour any map so that no neighbouring regions having non-point common boundaries get the same colour. This problem belongs to graph theory, a branch of mathematics. It was first proposed in 1840 by A F Möbius (1790–1868) and was proved to be correct in 1976 by Haken and Appel of the University of Illinois (USA) using 1200 hours of computer time to perform an extremely complex analysis involving a set of 1936 graphs.

Since the conjecture is proved, it is now the 4 colour theorem and no more a mere conjecture.

8.8 Fermat's Last Theorem (Theorem at Last)

The statement "The equation $x^n + y^n = z^n$ has no solution in integers with $xyz \neq 0$ for $n > 2$" is known as Fermat's last theorem. It was posed in 1637 by Fermat. Though it is called a theorem, it was really a conjecture till 1994 when it was proved by Andrew Wiles. Thus at last it really became a theorem [10].

8.9 Patterns and Conjectures

Observing patterns lead us to make conjectures. When we observe a pattern, we sometimes get a strong feeling that we have hit upon some hidden underlying property, which we believe, can be proved, though the proof does not occur to us immediately. Counter-examples also do not surface and we become bold enough to make a conjecture. But one has to be extremely cautious and careful, since sometimes a counter-example is just under our nose. We miss it because of our over-enthusiasm and are led to the trap of a wrong conjecture. We cite some examples of this type. Consider numbers of the form $2^{2^n}+1$. The resulting numbers are all primes for $n = 0, 1, 2, 3, 4$. From this observation, even the great Fermat ventured to conjecture that the integers of the form 2^{2^n} are primes. But he was wrong. Euler pointed out that even the very next number, namely $2^{2^5}+1$ is a composite, a product of 641 and $6,700,417$.

As another example, consider the sequence whose initial numbers are $31, 331, 3331, 33331, 333331, 3333331, 33333331$. All these are primes. But we will be conjecturing wrong, if by observing this pattern, we state that an integer starting with any number of 3s followed by 1 as the last digit, is a prime. The pattern that we observed above is what is called self-destructive as the number next in line to those given above, namely 333333331 is composite having factors 17 and $19,607,843$.

In attempts to find formulae to generate primes, many investigators hit upon self-destructive patterns. For example, numbers generated by the formula n^2+n+41 are primes for $n = 0, 1, 2, \ldots, 39$, while for $n = 40$ it produces a composite. Similarly $n^2 - 79^n + 1601$ yields primes for $n = 0, 1, 2, \ldots, 79$ and for $n = 80$, it generates a composite.

8.10 de Polignac's Conjecture

Around 1850, the French mathematician A de Polignac conjectured: "Every odd number can be expressed as the sum of a power of 2 and a prime." He claimed that he checked his assertion for all odd numbers up to 3 million. Since no positive power of 2 can have an odd number in its prime factorisation, had it been true, Polignac's assertion would have been a marvellous result. But alas, it is patently wrong. Polignac said that he verified his claim for many many numbers, but actually missed a simple counter-example, namely 127. Let us express 127 as a sum of a power of 2 and the remaining numbers in all possible ways:

$127 = 1 + 126 = 2^\circ + (9 \times 14) = 2 + 125 = 2 + (5 \times 25) = 4 + 123 = 2^2 + (3 \times 41) = 8 + 119 = 2^3 + (7 \times 17) = 16 + 111 = 2^4 + (3 \times 37) = 32 + 95 =$

$2^5 + (5 \times 19) = 64 + 63 = 2^6 + (7 \times 9)$. Since $2^7 = 128 > 127$, our verification is over; we see that the second component of 127 is not a prime in each case. So Polignac's conjecture is disproved.

8.11 Goldbach's Conjecture

Goldbach's conjecture, stated in 1742, says that every even integer greater than 4 can be expressed as a sum of two odd primes. Even though many of the ablest mathematicians have tried for more than two centuries and a half, this conjecture remains unsettled. But a weaker version of this conjecture, namely "A sufficiently large even number is the sum of a prime and an almost prime" has been proved by the Chinese mathematician Chen. [See Lecture 5, Section 5.4 and Lecture 10, Section 10.7]

8.12 Ramanujan's Hypothesis or Tau Conjecture

Let $\sigma_s(n)$ denote the sum of the sth powers of the divisors of n. If $n = 4$, its divisors are $1, 2, 4$. If $s = 2, \sigma_2(4) = 1^2 + 2^2 + 4^2 = 21$. In order to calculate $\sigma_s(n)$ generally, Ramanujan introduced the tau function, $\tau(n)$.

$\tau(n)$ is an arithmetical function. An arithmetical function is one that originates in trying to learn certain properties of numbers. Some other examples of arithmetical functions are $\pi(n)$, the number of prime numbers among the first n numbers, and $P(n)$, the number of partitions of the positive integer n.

Ramanujan conjectured that $\tau(n)$ is of the form $O(n^{\frac{11}{2}+\epsilon})$. Hardy called it Ramanujan's hypothesis. It is more generally known as the tau conjecture. It meant that the value of $\tau(n) \leq kn^{\frac{11}{2}+\epsilon}$ for some constant k, for all $n > n_0$ (say).

Ramanujan himself had proved that $\tau(n) = O(n^7)$. But the power 7 here, of n, is much more than $11/2$, and very much short of proving the conjecture. Two years later, Hardy came little closer to the proof when he proved $\tau(n) = O(n^6)$. Kloosterman got closer in 1927, Davenport and Salie still closer in 1933. The Scottish mathematician Robert Rankin, Hardy's student, proved in 1939, that $\tau(n) = O(n^{29/5})$. All this was somewhat like showing first that your friend lived at a house on MG Road number less than 1215; then, that the house number was less than 1201; then less than 1199... And yet one could still not establish that he/she lived at 1196, which is where the friend actually lived.

Finally, the Belgian mathematician Pierre Deligne proved the conjecture in 1974 using algebraic geometry. This is considered as one of the sparkling achievements of the 20th century. For this great achievement Deligne was awarded the Fields Medal, which is considered as the Nobel prize for mathematics.

8.13 Conjecture known as the Riemann Hypothesis

Zeta function is an infinite series expressed in terms of a complex variable. In 1860, Georg Friedrich Bernhard Riemann made six conjectures regarding the zeta function. By about 1920, five of them were proved right. The sixth is now known as the Riemann hypothesis.

The Riemann Hypothesis asserts that the non-trivial zeros of the Riemann zeta function lie on the line $x = 1/2$. This conjecture is rated as the deepest existing unsettled problem in pure mathematics. It implies that primes occur in a very subtle and precise pattern and not randomly. If the hypothesis is true, conclusions going beyond the prime number theorem would follow.

Around 1914, Hardy proved something short of the hypothesis. He proved that an infinite number of solutions of the zeta functions lie on $x = 1/2$. But that does not amount to saying that all did as claimed by the conjecture.

8.14 Ramanujan's Conjecture about the Partition Function

Integer 4 can be obtained from positive integers, using only addition, in 5 ways: $4; 3+1; 2+2; 2+1+1; 1+1+1+1$. These are called partitions of 4 and the fact is denoted as $P(4) = 5$. In general, $P(n)$, an arithmetical function, stands for the number of partitions of positive integer n.

Ramanujan's conjecture regarding this partition function is: "If $(24n - 1) = O \pmod{m^{\alpha}}$, where m is $5, 7$ or 11, and $\alpha \geq 1$, then $P(n) \equiv O(\text{mod } m^{\alpha})$". S Chawla showed that Ramanujan's conjecture failed for $n = 243$. For his proof, he used the table of partitions prepared by Hansraj Gupta [5]. Later it was also found that Ramanujan's conjecture failed for $n = 586$.

8.15 Conjecture that Came to be Known as the Prime Number Theorem

Let $\pi(x) =$ the number of primes less than or equal to the integer x. For example, $\pi(8) = 4$ since $2, 3, 5$ and 7 are the four primes less than or equal to 8. Similarly one can verify that $\pi(9) = \pi(10) = 4, \pi(13) = 6$. Again $\pi(10,00,000) = 78498, \pi(90,00,000) = 602,489$.

$\pi(x)/x$ will give the proportion of numbers less than or equal to x, that are primes. In the papers belonging to 14-year old Gauss, there appeared the following line: "Prime numbers below $a(= \infty)$ was approximately equal to a/la". This was the birth of the conjecture. In modern terminology, prime numbers below $a = \pi(a)$; "$a(= \infty)$" means "as $a \to \infty$" or "for large values of a;" "la" means "$\ln a$". Thus what Gauss wrote was $\pi(a) \approx a/\ln a$, for large values of a. This is the same thing as

$$\underset{a \to \infty}{\text{lt}} \frac{\pi(a)}{a} \approx \frac{1}{\ln a}$$

for large values of a. This is the prime number theorem as is stated these days. So Gauss recognised it, though he did not prove it. At last in 1896, the French mathematician, Jacques Hadamard (1865–1963), and the Beligian C J de la Vallé Poussin (1866–1962) proved the long-conjectured prime number theorem. They proved it independently and simultaneously.

Stated differently, the theorem says: $\pi(x) \ln x/x \to 1$ as $x \to \infty$. This approximation gives no clue to its accuracy; it does not specify how "fast" the ratio approaches 1.

Ramanujan, in his first letter to Hardy, had written: "I have found a function which exactly represents the number of prime numbers less than x". Actually he was mistaken, he had not found the correct function. Ramanujan's formula was an infinite series. He gave three versions of it in his second letter to Hardy. For values up to 1000, Ramanujan's formula virtually gave exact agreement. It was known that there were 602, 489 primes below nine million. Ramanujan's formula gave the figure off by just 53. This was better than the performance of the prime number theorem. Ramanujan relied too much on the low values of x for which he had tried his formula. The error for higher values of x was much larger than he thought. Hardy still found Ramanujan's approach very illuminating. He wrote: "Ramanujan's theory was what the theory might be if the zeta function had no complex zeros."

8.16 Word of Caution

Sometimes proofs are put forward to certify that a certain conjecture is right or wrong. Many times it is difficult to find a mistake in the proof or to say that the proof is correct. Sometimes mistakes lie undetected for quite a long time, as they are very subtle in nature. For example, a London lawyer Alfred Kempe (a former student of Cayley) published a proof of the four colour conjecture in 1879. Others also published alternative proofs. Kempe was honoured. Yet one day in 1890, P J Heawood identified a subtle mistake in Kempe's proof. Kempe admitted the gap in his reasoning. Other so-called proofs were demolished more easily and the problem returned to the status of a conjecture. But it took 11 years for the mistake to be pointed out. Similarly in 1988, a Japanese mathematician Yoichi Miyaoka, working at Princeton gave a proof of Fermat's last theorem. But a mistake was discovered in it within a few months during which period there was, naturally, a lot of excitement. The moral of all this is that one has to be ever cautious and careful [2].

Conclusions

We have acquainted ourselves with certain conjectures in the field of mathematics. Now taking advantage of the high speed and big storage available with computers, our capacity to experiment with mathematical objects has increased many-fold, making us equipped and competent to notice and verify various properties of these objects. This further enhances our ability to make surmises. Good knowledge, appreciation, and understanding of mathematics will be useful and necessary to prove or disprove these guesses. References [1] and [4] can help in this purpose.

Lecture 9

How Well do We Learn and Teach Mathematics?

Abstract

Standard stereotype examinations and the pressures brought on by them, partly due to heavy competiton and lack of peace and concentration of mind have caused one's preparations and studies for tests and examinations to become lopsided. The very essence of understanding the basic concepts properly is lost in the maze of details of computations. We bring out, with apt illustrations, some such happenings in the education of mathematics with the expectation that the concerned teachers and students pay due attention and improve the scenario for the benefit of all.

9.1 Introduction

A student of an engineering college once told me that in the course book of mathematics that he was asked to follow, the chapter on "Fourier Series" started as follows. After the title, a box contained the equation:

$$f(x) = \left(\frac{a_0}{2}\right) + \sum_{n=1}^{\infty} a_n \cos nx + \sum_{n=1}^{\infty} b_n \sin nx,\, a_n = \ldots,\, b_n = \ldots$$

Then below the box, various examples were solved by taking different functions like $f(x) = x^2$, $f(x) = x$, $\sin x$, etc., and finding out a_n and b_n in each case and then writing down $f(x)$ in its series form as above with the corresponding a_n and b_n. The student further said that he did not understand (even though he got very good marks and a good grade) why a_n and b_n should be calculated like that and what they represent, and further what the Fourier series stood for. He said that the situation was the same with every topic in the book.

There are many important points which need proper attention while learning and teaching mathematics [5, 6, 8]. I have decided to touch upon some of them here through simple examples, as simple examples convey the desired point sufficiently well. With my experience of teaching students who have obtained their bachelor's degree in either science or engineering, and in some cases, even with those who have obtained a master's degree, I have found that they have not properly assimilated these points. Therefore, I venture to emphasise them here.

9.2 Sequences

Consider first " sequences ". It is a common practice to ask a question of the following type: " What is the next term in the sequence $2, 4, 6, 8, \ldots ?$". I am sure that you must have asked such a question and/or seen such a question being asked in an examination. Most everybody would expect the answer to be 10. Suppose a student gives the answer 34. What would we do to him? I am afraid we would penalise him by giving zero or sometimes even negative marks for this answer. I regret it, but you might even call him/her a poor student of mathematics. But actually the student is also correct. If I ask, " Why is the next term in the given sequence 10?," I will get the following types of answers: " the difference between successive terms is 2", " the given terms are successive even integers", " the given terms are successive multiples of 2", " the general term which generates the given members of the sequence is $2n$". You think that you have recognised the general term, namely $2n$, correctly. But if we consider $n^4 - 10n^3 + 35n^2 - 48n + 24$ as a general term, we can see that putting $n = 1, 2, 3, 4$ respectively in it will give us $2, 4, 6, 8$ as the beginning terms of the sequence. And so it is perfectly legitimate to consider $n^4 - 10n^3 + 35n^2 - 48n + 24$ as a correct general term. Then putting $n = 5$ in it will yield 34 and that is why I said that 34 is also a correct answer.

The moral of this example is the fact that " a sequence cannot be defined by writing down its finite number of terms, however large that number of terms might be". If this fact is not understood and appreciated by a student, he/she would only give the answer 10 to our above question. In fact, any number of general terms like the two above (namely $2n$, and $n^4 - 10n^3 + 35n^2 - 48n + 24$) can be found which will generate $2, 4, 6, 8$ when $n = 1, 2, 3, 4$ are put in each of them. This means that there could be an infinite number of possible answers to the question posed. Hence it is really wrong to ask such a question. A particular answer being wrong or right apart, asking such a question gives a conceptually wrong impression to a student that he/she can specify a sequence by giving its finite number of terms. This misconception is a great stumbling block to his/her becoming a good student of mathematics. Since the two sequences $\{2n\}$, and $\{n^4 - 10n^3 + 35n^2 - 48n + 24\}$ are different, even though some of the initial terms of both are identical, a student should learn through his/her learning and studies that the only way to define a sequence is by defining its general term. Without the general term, a sequence is not defined. So really speaking $\{2, 4, 6, 8, \ldots\}$ is not a sequence at all. On the other hand, $\{2, 4, 6, 8, \ldots, 2n, \ldots\}$ or writing alternatively or simply $\{2n\}$ is a sequence. Similarly, $\{2, 4, 6, 8, \ldots, n^4 - 10n^3 + 35n^2 - 48n + 24, \ldots\}$ or $\{n^4 - 10n^3 + 35n^2 - 48n + 24\}$ is a sequence. This point must be emphasised.

You could possibly ask the question as: "What is the possible next term in the sequence whose first four terms are 2, 4, 6, 8? Why?", so that the student will give the general term and then only will deserve the marks due to him. We can also avoid the unnecessary penalisation of the student because we will know the general term that is on his mind.

When I discuss this in my lectures, I am asked as to how I got the general term, $n^4 - 10n^3 + 35n^2 - 48n + 24$. This expression has more higher degree terms than $2n$. Since $2n$ and $n^4 - 10n^3 + 35n^2 - 48n + 24$ produce the same values for $n = 1, 2, 3, 4$, to get the latter expression, we must add to $2n$, the terms which become zero for $n = 1, 2, 3, 4$. Obviously a possible term that gives zero for $n = 1, 2, 3, 4$ is given by $(n-1)(n-2)(n-3)(n-4)$. Therefore $2n + (n-1)(n-2)(n-3)(n-4)$ is a possible general term which yields $2, 4, 6, 8$ for $n = 1, 2, 3, 4$ respectively. When simplified, it gives the expression given above. Again $2n + \alpha(n-1)(n-2)(n-3)(n-4)$ will also serve the required purpose for any value of α. That is why, we stated above that infinite number of possible answers could be given to the question which we started with.

9.3 Functions

Now our next question is: "Describe clearly what is written below:

$$f(x) = x + 2, x = -1, 0, 1, 2,$$

$$g(x) = x^4 - 2x^3 - x^2 + 3x + 2, x = -1, 0, 1, 2\text{"}$$

The most common answer that I have obtained is: "You have written two functions." Sometimes if there is a smarter listener in the audience, he/she says: "You have written two different functions having the same domain." Even providing some extra time does not, generally, produce a better answer. But we can see that $f = \{(-1, 1), (0, 2), (1, 3), (2, 4)\} = g$. Thus if we remember that a function is a set of ordered pairs with the property that the first members of the ordered pairs are different, we should realise that what is written in the statement of the question is the same function in two different forms. When one comes across such a situation, one wonders whether the concept of a function itself, so basic to the whole tower of mathematics, is properly assimilated, understood and appreciated. Because of the frequent use of f, g, etc., to name the functions, the underlying concept is lost in the maze of details of notations used to name the various appearances of the concept. We know that a person remains the same person, even if he/she wears different dresses on different occasions. Similarly, a function is a fundamental concept; the same function can appear in different forms with different names, like f, g, h etc., and we should be able to recognise and identify them, if we want to be properly acquainted with them.

Further, it must be known that when we write $f(x)$, actually f is the function, though by abuse of language, we say function $f(x)$, which really is the value of f at x, just as $f(2)$ is the value of function f at value 2 of the concerned independent variable. As such, in modern notation, a function is specified as $f : A \to B$, where $x \to f(x)$, A and B are respectively domain and co-domain (or range) of the function f, and $f(x)$ is the concerned formula like $x + 2$ or the like.

9.4 Independence of Events

Consider now the concept of "independence of two events" that occurs when we study probability. If we ask the question: "When are two events A and B called independent?", many times, the reply is: "Two events A and B are called independent if the happening of one does not affect the happening of the other." Some books (not the good ones) too give such a definition. But it is not correct. If we look at another way of introducing the independence of two events, it will throw light on what I am saying. We say that the two events A and B are independent if $P(A) = P(A|B)$ and $P(B) \neq 0$ or $P(B) = P(B|A)$ and $P(A) \neq 0$. Note that $P(B|A)$ is called the conditional probability of B under the condition that event A has occured (or taken place or materialised). On the other hand, $P(B)$ is the unconditional probability of B. Thus two events A and B are called independent if the respective unconditional and conditional probabilities of one of the events are equal, or in other words, if the (unconditional) probability of one event is not affected (i.e., not changed) by the happening of the other. So we note, from this definition, critically that when two events are independent, what is not affected is the probability of the happening of one of them and not merely happening (which means physical happening) as stated in one definition given at the beginning by the occurence of the other.

As an example, suppose that two true (i.e., unbiased) coins are tossed one after another. Let A denote the event that the first coin shows head, and let B denote the event that the second coin shows head. Now we know that $P(B) = 1/2, P(B|A) = 1/2$. Hence the events A and B are independent. Note that the probability of the happening of B is not affected by the happening of A. It remains 1/2 when A happens or not. A does not happen means event not-A happens, i.e., the first coin does not show head, i.e., it shows tail. So the second coin will show head with probability 1/2 whether the first coin shows head or tail. The same situation will prevail whether one of the two or both the coins are biased – that is, the probability of the second coin showing head remains the same, whether the first coin shows head or tail.

Consider now the example of drawing two cards one after the other, from a well-shuffled pack of playing cards, without replacement. Let C stand for the event that the first card drawn is a red one, and let D stand for the event that the second card drawn is a black one. Now $P(D|C) = 26/51$, and $P(D) = 1/2$. Here $P(D) \neq P(D|C)$, and hence C and D are not independent events (i.e., they are dependent events). Note that it is the probability of the happening of D that is affected by the happening or not happening of C. It is not that the happening of C affects the physical happening of D, in the sense that if C happens, all the black cards disappear or the hands of the drawer are injured and the like.

Therefore, our first definition should be modified by introducing the word "probability" at the right place. Thus "two events A and B are called independent if the happening of one does not affect the *probability* of the happening of the other." The concept of the independence of events is based on the concept of probability and surprisingly there was no mention of the word probability in the definition given initially; we have now corrected that mistake.

Students should clearly understand and appreciate that the notion of independence of events cannot be introduced at all without knowing what "probability" means. In contrast to this the concept of mutually exclusive (i.e., disjoint) events can be introduced without the foreknowledge of the concept of probability.

9.5 Limitations of Methods

Periodically we update the syllabi of all subjects, and in particular, of mathematics at different levels. While doing so, we take into consideration the new discoveries in the subject, the applications that the existing and new knowledge have made possible, the new simple methods of presentation discovered, and the impact that discoveries in other related fields of knowledge might have made on our subject. Considering all these factors, we include, delete, expand, curtail and modify the various topics in our syllabi. For example, the contents of courses on Euclidean geometry have been modified in our syllabi at all levels. One factor that has made a great impact on mathematics in recent times is the advent of computers.The computer is, in fact, a child of applied mathematics. Our present students are going to be exposed to computers in all walks of their lives. We should consciously keep this in mind and try to bring the impact of computers in our teaching of mathematics. I do not mean at all that the working of computers and programming, in particular, computer languages should be a part of the syllabi in mathematics. But we should certainly modify or change certain aspects of the teaching of mathematics.

Let me explain this with an example. Consider a system of non-homogeneous, linear, independent, algebraic equations equal to the number of unknown variables, say three:

$$\sum_{j=1}^{3} a_{ij}x_j = b_i \, , i = 1, 2, 3, \tag{1}$$

We teach how the solution to (1) is given by $x_i = (\Delta_i/\Delta)(i = 1, 2, 3)$, where Δ is the determinant of the coefficient of x_is in (1), and Δ_i is Δ in which the ith column is replaced by RHS in (1). This is what is known as Cramer's rule. In the simple example given here, we have to evaluate determinants of 4 matrices, each of order 3. Each determinant is a sum of 3! terms, each term requiring 2 multiplications. Hence the solution of (1) needs $4 \times 3! \times 2 = 48$ multiplications plus 20 additions, and 3 divisions to be performed. When a student learns this method, he naturally expects it to be applicable to any number of such equations. If we want to solve a system of 20 such equations, using Cramer's rule, the solution will require $21 \times 20! \times 19$ multiplications, apart from additions and divisions. A reasonably modern computer performs $100,000$ multiplications per second. On this computer itself, the multiplications for the solution of 20 equations alone would require about 3×10^8 years, provided the computer does not breakdown part way through these calculations. Twenty equations of this type in 20 unknowns is not an unusual situation in practical problems. The student should know that Cramer's rule, if employed, would require more than 2 million years (even if a computer capable of performing 2 million operations per second, and running continuously is used) to solve a system of 20 equations in 20 unknowns. And he should know it right when he is studying this method, rather than knowing it sometime later. What we have done above is to analyse Cramer's rule in terms of the total number of basic operations it requires. A student should be taught to carry out such analysis of any algorithm right at the time of his learning that algorithm so that he/she knows the advantages and limitations of every method as and when he studies that method. Otherwise there is a great chance that he/she may get a shock when she attempts to solve a practical problem using that method and gets bogged down by its limitations.

9.6 Definition of a Matrix

When we ask what a matrix is, students from high schools to post-graduate classes invariably say that it is a rectangular arrangement of entities. An $m \times n$ matrix has mn entries; these positions can be specified by $\{(i, j), i = 1, 2, ., m, j = 1, 2, \ldots, n\}$. At each of these positions, we specify a certain definite entity. From this description, it should be clearly evident that we can define an $m \times n$ matrix as a function where domain is the cross-product $M \times N$, where $M = \{1, 2, \ldots, m\}$ and $N = \{1, 2, \ldots, n\}$. In a sequence, a similar situation exists, except that we have a linear arrangement of its members, rather than a rectangular one as in matrices. When students are taught that a sequence can be defined as a function whose domain is $N = \{1, 2, 3, \ldots\}$, the set of natural numbers, why not similarly define a matrix as a function, as described above? Would not that be more mathematical? Students can and should be told that a rectangular arrangement is just one possible representation of the mathematical object known as matrix. A representation should not be confused with the definition.

9.7 Definition of Determinant

Just as in the case of matrix, it will not do if we define a determinant in terms of its representation by saying that it is a square arrangement of numbers put between two vertical bars. Notation of vertical bars or brackets should not be used to distinguish between the definition of a determinant and that of a matrix. These are after all concepts, and the essence of the concept should get reflected in the definition of that concept, rather than relying on the method of representation.

Matrix is not a number; it is a new entity like sequence or vector. On the other hand, determinant is a number with which we are acquainted from the beginning of our study of mathematics. Number 2.1 can be represented in various ways as

$$2\frac{1}{10}, \frac{42}{20}, 21 \times 10^{-1}, 0.21 \times 10^{1} \text{ or as a determinant.}$$

$$\begin{vmatrix} 2.1 & 3.5 \\ 4.2 & 8 \end{vmatrix}$$

To come up with a good mathematical definition of a determinant, let us examine the expansion of a 3×3 determinant:

$$\begin{vmatrix} a_{11} & a_{12} & a_{13} \\ a_{21} & a_{22} & a_{23} \\ a_{31} & a_{32} & a_{33} \end{vmatrix} = a_{11}a_{22}a_{33} - a_{11}a_{23}a_{32} + a_{12}a_{23}a_{31}$$
$$-a_{12}a_{21}a_{33} + a_{13}a_{21}a_{32} - a_{13}a_{22}a_{31}$$

We observe the following properties of this expansion:

i. The first suffixes of the elements in each of the six terms are in natural order, i.e., 1, 2, 3.
ii. The second suffixes of the elements in each term is a permutation of 1, 2, 3.
iii. A term has a positive or negative sign if the second suffixes of the elements in that term form an even permutation or odd permutation, respectively, of 1, 2, 3.
iv. In each term, each digit from the digits 1, 2, 3 occurs once and only once, as a first suffix as well as a second suffix; there is no repetition of any suffix.
v. Order 3 of the determinant gives its number of rows as well as number of columns.
vi. The total number of terms $= 3! = 6 =$ total number of permutations of the three numbers 1, 2, 3.

If we think about and reflect on these properties of the determinant of order n, we can come up with the following definition by generalisation:

A determinant of order n is given by

$$\sum_{i_1=1}^{n}\sum_{i_2=1}^{n}\cdots\sum_{i_{n1}=1}^{n} e_{i_1 i_2\ldots i_n}\, a_{1i_1}a_{2i_2}\ldots a_{ni_n}$$

where $e_{i_1 i_2\ldots i_n} = +1$ if $i_1 i_2 \ldots i_n$ is an even permutation of $1, 2, \ldots n$,

$= -1$ if $i_1 i_2 \ldots i_n$ is an odd permutation of $1, 2, \ldots n$,

$= 0$ otherwise.

The real import of the concept of determinant will not be understood unless we define it as above. We can easily tell from this definition (using our knowledge of permutations), that a determinant of order n, when expanded, contains $n!$ terms (generally, students are not able to state this in their answers).

9.8 Definitions in General—Their Meaning

Normally a study of a new topic in mathematics starts with some definitions. Thus definitions occupy an extremely important position and play a very significant role in our learning and teaching of mathematics. I want to bring out an aspect of a definition that is normally missed by students. Let us start with a simple example. If we ask any student to define an equilateral triangle, he/she will correctly answer as follows: "A triangle is called equilateral, if all its sides are equal". Let me state positively that the student is correct in his/her definition. But it will be clear from the following discussion that most students have not understood an important aspect of such definitions. After he/she gives the above-stated definition, I can argue with the student as follows: "The definition says that if all the sides of a triangle are equal, then the triangle is called equilateral. But if you are told, that a triangle ABC is equilateral, can you conclude that all its sides are equal?" He/she may answer in the affirmative. I can continue arguing with him/her as follows: "But your definition does not permit you to do so. It only tells you that if all its sides are equal, then the triangle is equilateral. It does not say that if the triangle is equilateral, then all its sides are equal." The student appreciates the argument and has no answer. He fumbles as the situation is different from his usual experience. Whenever he/she has been given a triangle that is equilateral, he/she has automatically taken it for granted that all its sides are equal on the basis of the definition only and nobody had objected. Hence he/she is surprised to hear such a question in discussion on the meaning of an equilateral triangle's definition. All this has happened because neither has it occured in his/her mind any time while learning, nor have his/her teachers brought it to his attention any time while teaching that the definition really is: "If all the sides of a triangle are equal, then it is called equilateral and if a triangle is known to be equilateral, then all its sides are equal" or equivalently "*A triangle is called equilateral if and only if (iff) all its sides are equal*". What is important to note is that such is the situation with all the definitions that include the word "if" (note that every definition explicitly or implicitly includes the word "if"). Therefore it is an accepted convention in mathematics that the appearance of "if and only if" in a definition, is replaced by merely "if".

I would say that one has not understood any definition correctly and fully if one does not know the above-explained meaning of the word "if" in definitions. Hence it should be emphasised duly. In fact, this aspect could be profitably utilised to neatly explain with the help of simple examples, the equivalence of the phrases "if and only if", "necessary and sufficient condition", "such and such and conversely", and the notation "$\Leftrightarrow$". The definition of an equilateral triangle can be stated using any of these ways. We have already used "iff" above. Other usages will give us the following alternative statements of the definitions:

"*The necessary and sufficient condition for a triangle to be equilateral is that all its sides are equal.*"

"*A triangle is called equilateral if all its sides are equal and conversely.*"
"*A triangle is equilateral* $\Leftrightarrow$ *all its sides are equal*".

In a general case, we know that the converse is not always true. But it is always true in the case of a definition involving the word "if", since "if" in definition connotes "if and only if". Since the converse is always true for a definition, there is no point in mentioning so with every definition. That is the reason why "iff" in a definition is replaced by just "if" as a routine. This should be clearly understood while learning, and should be properly brought out while teaching. It is all the more important because a particular quality that distinguishes mathematics from other subjects in the syllabi is its particular emphasis on logical consequence. The characteristic statement of mathematics is "If A, then B"

9.9 Definitions—Particular and General

Let us turn to another aspect of definitions. As we develop the subject in book, in notes, or in a class, we often initially give a definition applicable to a simple and restricted situation and then generalise it. When we ask a student to define such a term, I feel we should expect from him the generalised definition subject to his/her level of study at that time. Let me illustrate this, again, with a simple example of common occurence. If we ask for the formula for ${}^nC_r$, we would most probably get the answer $n!/[r!(n-r)!]$. We all know that this is true only if n and r are non-negative integers. We also know that the concept of ${}^nC_r$ is generalised further to cover negative and fractional values of n and is used in the negative binomial theorem. In that case, the formula is ${}^nC_r = n(n-1)(n-2)\dots(n-r+1)/r!$ We note that in any case r is restricted to a non-negative integer only. When we ask a question calling for a definition or a formula as an answer, it is but natural to expect an answer that will be applicable in the most general manner possible. Thus it is imperative that one should encourage a student to state the formula $n(n-1)(n-2)\dots(n-r+1)/r!$, if he has learnt it, rather than the formula $n!/[r!(n-r)!]$ if he is asked to give one for ${}^nC_r$. The former formula subsumes the latter, i.e., it gives the same answer which the latter gives and is applicable for values of n for which the latter becomes meaningless.

Here a student may wonder why mathematicians have not derived a formula for ${}^nC_r$ when r is negative or fractional, when they have such a formula for when n is fractional or negative. We can take this opportunity to tell students that there is no situation where ${}^nC_r$ is useful or applicable if r is negative or fractional. On the other hand, the formula for ${}^nC_r$, when n is negative or fractional is useful, for example, in binomial theorem. We can supplement this information by telling students that there is no division in vectors even though division operation exists in real numbers. Similarly, there are two multiplication operations in vectors, while there is only one among numbers. In mathematics, operations or formulae are introduced only when they are called for from the applicability point of view.

We shall site some more examples of this type just to emphasise the point of view under discussion. We define the gamma function by an integral as $\Gamma(n) = \int_0^\infty e^{-x}x^{n-1}dx$ for $n > 0$. From this definition, we establish the property $\Gamma(n) = (n-1)\Gamma(n-1)$ and then use this property as a definition of $T(n)$ for non-integral negative values of n. If a student is asked to give a definition of gamma function, we should expect an answer that will be applicable to all possible values of n.

In probability theory, the definition of independence of two events can be given as:

"*Events A and B are called independent if P (A) = P (A | B).*"

But this definition is valid only if $P(B) \neq 0$, because this requirement is embodied in the definition of $P(A|B)$, which is $P(A|B) = P(AB)|P(B), P(B) \neq 0$. A better definition which does not impose this restriction is: "*Events A and B are called independent if P(AB)=P(A).P(B).*" This latter definition should be given, if somebody asks you to define "independence of two events" as it is applicable in all situations without any restriction like $P(B) \neq 0$.

Similarly, the definition "vector is an element of a vector space" brings matrices, functions etc into the fold of the term "vector". A student who has learnt vector space, should state this general definition, when asked to define the term vector, rather than state "a vector is an entity which requires for its complete description, direction along with magnitude."

9.10 Definitions—Qualitative and Quantitative

When we introduce a new concept, initially, we want students to appreciate the motivation for introducing the concept. Hence we explain it through various examples and then give a definition which may be descriptive or qualitative. We then build up a quantitative definition. Quantitative definitions are useful in making calculations and in further development of the subject.

Let us again take the example of ^nC_r. Initially we state that ^nC_r is the number of ways of choosing r objects from n distinct objects. This statement gives the physical, i.e., practical interpretation of ^nC_r and can be considered as a qualitative definition of ^nC_r. Then we develop the formulae $^nC_r = n!/[r!(n-r)!] = n(n-1)(n-2)\ldots.(n-r+1)/r!$ as stated, in the previous section, and use the latter expression as the definition of ^nC_r to accommodate any rational value of n. This becomes therefore the quantitative definition of ^nC_r. As is evident, the qualitative definition is not useful to compute the values of ^nC_r, while the quantitative definition is. Therefore a student should be encouraged to give a quantitative definition in preference to qualitative definition, when he/she is asked to define any term.

Let us cite another example. The definition of two independent events first given in probability theory, while explaining the situation is: " Two events are said to be independent if the happening of one does not affect the probability of the happening of the other ". This is a qualitative definition and does not help us to decide whether two given events are independent. After giving the above qualitative definition, we develop the following quantitative definition through the use of the definition of conditional probability: " *Two events A and B are said to be independent if* $P(AB) = P(A).P(B)$ ". This can be employed to determine whether two given events D and E are independent or not, by computing the probabilities $P(D)$, $P(E)$ and $P(DE)$. Stating the initially given qualitative definition, when asked to define the independence of two events, and not the quantitative definition developed afterwards is like a college student singing a nursery rhyme when he/she is asked to recite a poem.

9.11 Computing Functional Values

Students calculate the values of many functions at different values of the independent variable. This leads them to think that values of any function can be computed for any value of its independent variable. This is a wrong impression and can be dispelled if we present the following simple example:

$$\begin{aligned} f(n) &= 1, \text{if there is a run of exactly } n \text{ 3s in the decimal expansion of } \pi \\ &= 0, \text{otherwise.} \end{aligned}$$

Decimal expansion of π is infinitely long. For concreteness suppose a run of exactly 500 3s does not exist at all in the decimal expansion of π. In that case we go on and on examining decimal expansion of π with the hope of getting the run of exactly 500 3s. This examination will not stop any time, and hence we will not be able to decide the value of $f(500)$. This example will serve as an eye-opener and will open the interesting and important topic of computable and non-computable functions, a pioneering field in mathematics.

9.12 What Does Prob (A) = 0 Convey?

If we ask the question " What does Prob $(A) = 0$ mean? ", we most probably will get the answer, " A is an impossible event ". But that is not true. Consider a circular disc (Fig. 9.1) which is calibrated between 0 and 100. 100 coincides with zero. At the centre of the disc, there is an elastic pointer. If we push the pointer, it rotates for a sufficiently long time, and finally stops.

Prob [the pointer will stop between 10 and 20] = 10/100.

Prob [the pointer will stop between 10 and 15] = 5/100.

Prob [the pointer will stop between 10 and 11] = 1/100.

Prob [the pointer will stop between 10 and 10.2]= 0.2/100, . . .,

and finally

Prob [the pointer will stop at 10] = 0.

Does this mean that the pointer will never stop at 10? No. The same is true for the pointer stopping at any particular point. This shows that Prob $(A) = 0$ indicates that A is very very rare or an "almost impossible" event, as it is called i.e. $[P(A) = 0] \Rightarrow A$ is an impossible event.

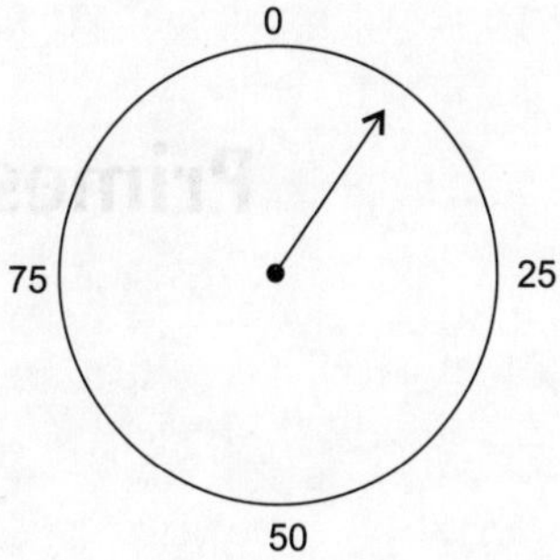

Fig. 9.1

Conclusion

Only if we emphasise conceptual and understanding aspects, along with calculational aspects, will the students be properly prepared for the challenging developmental work that they will be facing in their future lives in the rapidly changing world of today and tomorrow.

Lecture 10

Primes and Composites

Abstract

In our study of mathematics, we deal with different types of numbers. But primes and non-primes (i.e., composites) occupy a place of pride and honour. They also play a very precious role among all numbers. Here we will acquaint ourselves with some behaviour patterns of these types of numbers which have pleased the minds of many amateur and professional mathematicians – many of them who have spent a good part of their careers in studying them. Till recently this part of mathematics was considered the purest in the realm of the whole of mathematics.

10.1 Introduction

Everybody knows numbers. There are various ways of naming numbers. Some are called triangular numbers; some are perfect numbers; some are called friendly numbers; some are called demlo numbers, and the list goes on. But of all such ways of naming numbers, the most important and productive way is that of calling certain numbers as prime numbers or simply primes.

A natural number (or which is the same, a positive integer) greater than 1 is called prime if it has no factors other than 1 and the number itself. This definition can be paraphrased in another way as follows. A natural number greater than 1 is called prime if it cannot be written as a product of two smaller natural numbers. A natural number other than 1 is called a composite number or simply composite, if it is not a prime. Number 1 is neither prime nor composite. Thus $2, 5, 29$ are examples of primes, while $6, 28, 500$ are examples of composites. We shall study here some interesting but less mentioned properties of primes and composites.

One of the greatest mathematicians of all times, Carl Friedrich Gauss (1777–1855) wrote in his book *Disquisitiones Arithmeticae* (1801): "The problem of distinguishing prime numbers from composite numbers and of resolving the latter into their prime factors is known to be one of the most important and useful in arithmetic".

In some contexts, negative counterparts of primes, viz., $-2, -3, -5, \ldots$ etc., are also regarded as primes.

10.2 Strings of Composites

If we examine positive integers, we will notice that $24, 25, 26, 27$ and 28 is a string of 5 consecutive composites. This is not a one-off phenomena. There exists a systematic general formula for constructing such a string, as long as we like, of consecutive composites. Let us approach the formula by first giving specific examples. The formula gives $6! + 2 = 722, 6! + 3 = 723, 6! + 4 = 724, 6! + 5 = 725$, and $6! + 6 = 726$ as another string of five consecutive composites. Note that 2 is a factor of both 6! and 2. Hence $6! + 2$ is not a prime but a composite. Similarly, 3 is a factor of both 6! and 3, making 6! + 3, a composite. Similar arguments show that $6! + 4, 6! + 5$ and $6! + 6$ are composite numbers. Using the formula again, we get $902! + 2, 902! + 3, \ldots, 902! + 902$ as a string of 901 consecutive composites. From these two examples, it should be clear that the general formula giving a string of n consecutive composites is:

$$(n+1)! + 2, (n+1)! + 3, \ldots, (n+1)! + (n+1).$$

It should also be clear that one can construct a string of arbitrarily long length, of consecutive composites.

10.3 How Many Primes in all?

The above-mentioned procedure of generating as many consecutive composites as one desires, can give us a feeling that we can have as big a gap as we like between two primes, and hence even though there could be plenty of primes, the totality of primes is limited. But it turns out that an infinite number of primes exist. This fact can be established using the age-old Euclid's proof – by contradiction.

Alternatively, we have a theorem which states "between the whole numbers n and $2n$ (for any n) there must always lie at least one prime". The truth of the infinity of primes can be established immediately, using this theorem. Incidentally, it is interesting to note that this theorem regarding the existence of at least one prime between n and $2n$ $(n > 1)$ was proved by the Russian mathematician Chebycheff about a century ago, but his proof was very complicated. It was again proved in a simpler way during the 20th century by Paul Erdös (1913–2000), the Hungarian mathematician, when he was just 17.

10.4 Formula to Generate Primes

Even though the number of primes is infinite, many feel that we can still tame them and handle them more easily if we had a formula which would give all primes or a formula which gives only primes [6]. It is generally assumed by many that no such formula exists. But that is not true. The required formula indeed exists. It can be established that the function

$$f(x,y) = \frac{y-1}{2}\left[|B^2-1| - (B^2-1)\right] + 2, \tag{1}$$

where $B = x(y+1) - (y!+1)$, x, y being natural numbers, generates only primes, every prime, and each odd prime exactly once, though it does produce prime 2 most of the time.

10.5 Other Attempts for Finding a Formula and the Impossibility of a One-Variable Formula

Equation (1) is not the only formula for generating primes – though it is the most general one. Many have attempted to derive formulae for this and they have succeeded in a limited range. In 1772 Euler pointed out that the formula

$$g(n) = n^2 - n + 41$$

gives primes when $n = 1, 2, \ldots 40$. This is of course true; further it is interesting to note that if we take the formula

$$f(n) = n^2 + n + 41$$

it also gives primes for $n = 0, 1, 2, \ldots, 39$ and yields the same primes for $n = -1, -2, \ldots, -40$ since

$$f(0) = f(-1), f(1) = f(-2), \ldots, f(39) = f(-40).$$

Thus n^2+n+41 yields primes for 80 consecutive integers $x = -40, -39, \ldots, 38, 39$. Alternatively the function

$$p(n) = n^2 - 79n + 1601$$

gives the very primes (namely, those generated by the above-mentioned functions $g(n)$ and $f(n)$), for $n = 0, 1, 2, \ldots, 79$.

The computer MANIAC II has found that for the primes under 10 million, Euler's formula $n^2 + n + 41$ generated primes 47.5% of the time. For values of n below 2398, this formula has 50% probability of getting a prime. For values between 1 and 100, this formula yields 86 primes and only 14 composites (these being for the values $40, 41, 44, 49, 56, 65, 76, 81, 82, 84, 87, 89, 91,$ and 96 of n).

Another formula, like that of Euler's is given by Stanislaw Ulam and his colleagues: $q(n) = 4n^2 + 170n + 1847$. Its success rate is 46.6% and it generates 760 primes below 10 million that are not generated by Euler's formula.

One more such formula is $\phi(n) = 4n^2 + 4n + 59$, whose success rate is 43.7%. It generates 1500 primes not generated by Euler's $f(n)$ or Ulam's formulae $q(n)$ given above. Formula (1) that produces only primes, and each odd prime exactly once is a two-variable formula. One would prefer a one-variable formula for this purpose like Euler's or Ulam's. But the sad news is that mathematicians have proved that no formula even vaguely resembling Euler's can produce all the primes or nothing but primes.

10.6 Square Spirals and Primes

In one of his aimless scribbling in 1963, Ulam (the brilliant mathematician who did pioneering work on the atom bomb at Los Alamos) drew, starting with 1, a square spiral as shown in Fig. 10.1 [3]. To his surprise, as well as ours, the primes tended to fall on diagonal lines. We have encircled the odd primes to show you the pattern.

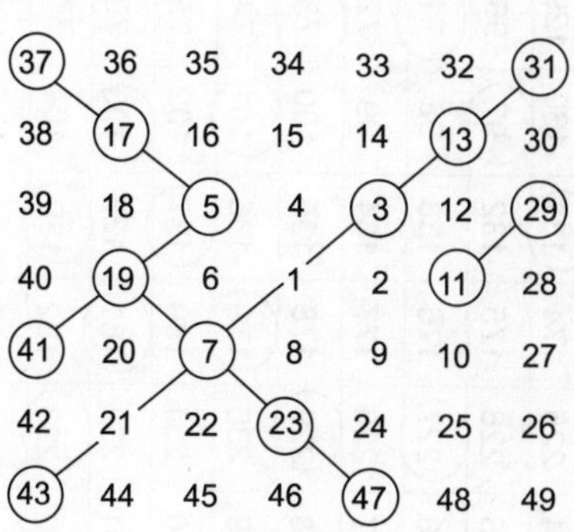

Fig. 10.1

Encouraged by the pattern displayed by the square spiral of Fig. 10.1, Ulam, Mark Wells and Myron Stein studied such square spirals starting with whole numbers other than 1. Figure 10.2 [3] gives one such square

421	420	**419**	418	417	416	415	414	413	412	411	410	**409**	408	407	406	405	404	403	402
422	**347**	346	345	344	343	342	341	340	339	338	**337**	336	335	334	333	332	**331**	330	**401**
423	348	**281**	280	279	278	**277**	276	275	274	273	272	**271**	270	**269**	268	267	266	329	400
424	**349**	282	**223**	222	221	220	219	218	217	216	215	214	213	212	**211**	210	265	328	399
425	350	**283**	224	**173**	172	171	170	169	168	**167**	166	165	164	**163**	162	209	264	327	398
426	351	284	225	174	**131**	130	129	128	**127**	126	125	124	123	122	161	208	**263**	326	**397**
427	352	285	226	175	132	**97**	96	95	94	93	92	91	90	121	160	207	262	325	396
428	**353**	286	**227**	176	133	98	**71**	70	69	68	**67**	66	**89**	120	159	206	261	324	395
429	354	287	228	177	134	99	72	**53**	52	51	50	65	88	119	158	205	260	323	394
430	355	288	**229**	178	135	100	**73**	54	**43**	42	49	64	87	118	**157**	204	259	322	393
431	356	289	230	**179**	136	**101**	74	55	44	**41**	48	63	86	117	156	203	258	321	392
432	357	290	231	180	**137**	102	75	56	45	46	**47**	62	85	116	155	202	**257**	320	391
433	358	291	232	**181**	138	**103**	76	57	58	**59**	60	**61**	84	115	154	201	256	319	390
434	**359**	292	**233**	182	**139**	104	77	78	**79**	80	81	82	**83**	114	153	200	255	318	**389**
435	360	**293**	234	183	140	105	106	**107**	108	**109**	110	111	112	**113**	152	**199**	254	**317**	388
436	361	294	235	184	141	142	143	144	145	146	147	148	149	150	**151**	198	253	316	387
437	362	295	236	185	186	187	188	189	190	**191**	192	**193**	194	195	196	**197**	252	315	386
438	363	296	237	238	**239**	240	**241**	242	243	244	245	246	247	248	249	250	**251**	314	385
439	364	297	298	299	300	301	302	303	304	305	306	**307**	308	309	310	**311**	312	**313**	384
440	365	366	**367**	367	369	370	371	372	**373**	374	375	376	377	378	**379**	380	381	382	**383**

Fig. 10.2

spiral starting with 41. In this also, we notice that primes tend to fall on diagonals. In particular, all the 20 entries on the principal diagonal are primes (421 through 383) and they are produced by Euler's formula $n^2 + n + 41$.

With the availability of computers, experimentation and enumeration of patterns has become comparatively easy and time-saving. In 1963, the MANIAC II mainframe computer at Los Alamos was used to store the first 90 million primes. It was also used to draw a square spiral diagram for all primes below 10 million and in that many primes were located on its diagonal lines.

10.7 Almost Prime Numbers

An integer is called an " almost prime " if it is a product of two primes. Thus the number 55 is almost prime, since $55 = 5 \times 11$, and 5 and 11 are primes. But 105 is not an almost prime since $105 = 3 \times 5 \times 7$, a product of three primes (and not two).

A theorem in prime number theory states that a sufficiently large even number is the sum of a prime and an almost prime. This was proved by the Chinese mathematician Chan. The theorem occupies such a vital place in prime number theory that Chan's proof is considered to be the most significant contribution to this field. The phrase " sufficiently large " in the statement of this theorem means " the proof (or the theorem) is true for all numbers greater than some number N, but what N is, is not known ". This may sound vague to a layman, but mathematically it is a perfectly sound phrase. For example, we say " divide the cylinder in sufficiently thin slices ", in applied mathematics while establishing certain results. Again " sufficiently thin " conveys that " every slice will have a thickness smaller than some value δ; the exact value of δ is not known but a thickness value smaller than δ is not necessary for the proof of the result. "

The above theorem proved by Chan is a weaker version of what is known as Goldbach's, conjecture (1742) given in Lecture 5, Section 5.4 which states, " every even number greater than 2 is the sum of two primes. " Christian Goldbach was a Prussian-born mathematician. Using computers, this conjecture is verified to be true for all even numbers up to 100 million. Many of the ablest mathematicians have tried their hands at this conjecture but without success.

10.8 Twin Primes and Triplet Primes

Primes of the form p and $p + 2$ are called twin primes. From among the primes between 1 and 100 (which are 25 in number), we have 8 pairs of twin primes. They are $(3, 5)$,$(5, 7)$,$(11, 13)$,$(17, 19)$, $(29, 31)$,$(41, 43)$,$(59, 61)$, and (71, 73). Among the primes between 101 and 200 (which are 21 in number), the twin primes are (101, 103), (107, 109), (137, 139), (149, 151), (179, 181), (191, 193), (197, 199). Among the large numbers (1, 000, 000, 000, 061; 1, 000, 000, 000, 063) is a twin prime pair.

There is a strong feeling among prime number theorists that twin primes are infinite in number. But this has not been proved yet. So it is not yet settled whether pairs of twin primes are finite or infinite, although Chan has proved a weaker result. The result is that there exist infinitely many pairs of numbers which differ by two in which the first number of the pair is a prime and the second is either a prime or an almost prime.

Primes of the form $p, p+2$, and $p+4$ are called triplet primes. In this case, it has been proved that there is only one prime triplet, namely (3, 5, 7).

10.9 Fundamental Theorem of Arithmetic

Our study of mathematics in primary school starts with arithmetic. Under arithmetic, we study integers and basic operations of addition, subtraction, multiplication, and division on them. Here too we are studying arithmetic – albeit special types of integers, namely, primes and composites, and some deeper properties of these numbers. This is somewhat harder than basic school arithmetic. Hence Europeans earlier called this subject, consisting of the extension of basic arithmetic, as "higher arithmetic". Nowadays it is known as "number theory". Often, the terms "arithmetic", "higher arithmetic", and "number theory" are used interchangeably.

It has been proved that every positive integer can be expressed as a product of its factors which are primes. For example, $360 = 2 \times 2 \times 2 \times 3 \times 3 \times 5 = 2^3.3^2.5$. Further, it is easy to appreciate that this prime factorisation can be done in one and only one way if we ignore the order in which the prime factors are enumerated. These facts are stated as: "*Any positive integer, other than 1 can be factorised into the product of primes uniquely (up to the order of primes)*". This theorem is known as the fundamental theorem of arithmetic. But for this theorem, primes, perhaps, would not have occupied such a central position in "arithmetic", or to use a more prestigious and sophisticated name, "number theory". This theorem shows that primes are the building blocks of numbers.

Conventionally, while expressing factors of any integer, primes are enumerated in the order of their magnitude, i.e., in the order 2, 3, 5, 7, 11, 13, 17, ... Thus any number N will be written, in terms of its prime factors, as

$$N = 2^{b_2}3^{b_3}.5^{b_5}.7^{b_7}.11^{b_{11}}\ldots.$$

To have a shorter notation, let $p_i = i$th prime, so that $p_1 = 2, p_2 = 3, p_3 = 5, p_4 = 7, p_5 = 11, p_6 = 13, p_7 = 17$, etc. Then the above N can be written as

$$N = p_1^{a_1}, p_2^{a_2} p_3^{a_3} \ldots = \prod_{i=1}^{\infty} p_i^{a_i}$$

(letting $b_2 = a_1, b_3 = p_1$, etc).

10.10 Divisors – their Number, Evenness, and Sum

Now we state some important and useful results based on prime factorisation of a number. If $N(>1)$ is a positive integer,

such that $N = \prod_{i-1}^{\infty} p_i^{a_1}$, then

- The total number of divisors (factors) of N
  $= \prod_{i=1}^{\infty} (a_i + 1)$
- The total numbers of divisors of N is odd if N is a perfect square, and even if N is not a perfect square
- Sum of all the divisors of N
  $= \prod_{i=1}^{\infty} \frac{p_i^{a_i+1} - 1}{p_i - 1}$

  Let us verify these results for some numbers:

1. $N = 24$. Its factors are $\{1, 2, 3, 4, 6, 8, 12, 24\}$. They are even (8) in number, and their sum is $1 + 2 + 3 + 4 + 6 + 8 + 12 + 24 = 60$. We have done these calculations in a direct way. Now by our above-mentioned formulae, since $24 = 2^3 \times 3$,

   total number of factors of $24 = (3 + 1) \times (1 + 1) = 8$,

   total number of factors must be even, as 24 is not a perfect square; and

   $$\text{sum of all factors of } 24 = \frac{2^4 - 1}{2 - 1} \times \frac{3^2 - 1}{3 - 1} = \frac{15}{1} \times \frac{8}{2} = 60.$$

   Thus the results obtained by direct calculations agree with those given by the use of the formulae, as expected.

2. $N = 36$. Its factors are $\{1, 2, 3, 4, 6, 9, 12, 18, 36\}$. The number of factors is odd (9), and their sum $= 1 + 2 + 3 + 4 + 6 + 9 + 12 + 18 + 36 = 91$.

This is by direct calculations. Now $36 = 2^2 \times 3^2$ and so using our formula

total number of factors of $36 = (2 + 1)(2 + 1) = 9$;

which is odd, and therefore 36 is a perfect square ($36 = 6^2$), and

$$\text{sum of all its divisors} = \frac{2^3 - 1}{2 - 1} \times \frac{3^3 - 1}{3 - 1} = \frac{7}{1} \times \frac{26}{2} = 91$$

Thus here also the results obtained by both the methods tally.

10.11 Highly Composite Numbers

Ramanujan, the most renowned Indian mathematical genius and highly rated mathematician of the 20th century, worked on prime numbers apart from other topics. He introduced what are known as "highly composite numbers" [5]. A composite number is known as highly composite number if the number of its divisors is more than those of any other smaller composite number. For example, composite number 24 has 8 divisors (as enumerated in Section 10.10), and this number 8 is more than the number of divisors of any of the composite numbers $4, 6, 8, 9, 10, 12, 14, 15, 16, 18, 20, 21$, and 22, each of them being smaller than 24. Therefore by definition, 24 is a highly composite number. On the other hand, 45 is a composite but not a highly composite number. This is so because 45 has in all 6 divisors, viz., $\{1, 3, 5, 9, 15, 45\}$ but a smaller composite number 24 has more divisors, viz., 8 as seen above. Ramanujan, in the first few pages of his second notebook listed about 100 highly composite numbers; the first few of them are $4, 6, 12, 24, 36, 48, 60, 120$.

Hardy, who can be called Ramanujan's mentor, aptly described a highly composite number by the phrase "as unlike a prime as a number can be".

Ramanujan discovered an important property of highly composite numbers. When one writes the prime factors of a natural number $N (> 1)$ as $N = 2^{b_2} 3^{b_3} 5^{b_5} \ldots$, b_2 will always be equal to or larger than b_3, b_3 will always be equal to or larger than b_5 and so on, if N is a highly composite number. For example, 24 is a highly composite number and $24 = 2^3 \times 3^1$; as such, indices of successive primes, starting from the first prime 2, form a non-increasing sequence. Note that in the prime factorisation $2^3 \times 3^1$ of 24, the indices of primes $5, 7, 11, \ldots$ are all zero and in line with the property stated above. The number 45 is not a highly composite number and so we do not expect this property to hold for it: $45 = 2^0 3^2 5^1$; index of 2 (zero) is smaller than that of 3 and the property is violated. Again $20 = 2^2 3^0 5^1$: here $b_2 > b_3$ but $b_3 < b_5$ and the property is violated as expected, since 20 is not a highly composite number. We would never find a highly composite number of the form $N = 2^5.3^6$ or of the form $M = 2^3.5^2 (= 2^3.3^0.5^2)$.

Ramanujan actually listed highly composite numbers up to a 13-digit number having 10080 factors. But in 1926 T. Vijayraghvan pointed out that Ramanujan had erred in that his list did not include a 12-digit highly composite number $293, 318, 625, 600$, which had 5040 factors.

Ramanujan also showed that with two exceptions (namely 4 and 36), the last b_n necessary to obtain a highly composite number is always 1. One can verify this with every composite number listed above. For example, $120 = 2^3.3.5$; here $b_2 = 3$, $b_3 = b_5 = 1$, ie., the last b_n is b_5 which is 1.

It is instructive to note that Ramanujan received his BA from the Cambridge University (UK) in March 1916 on the basis of his long paper on highly composite numbers.

10.12 Mersenne and Primes

Marin Mersenne (1588–1648) was a French priest with a love for numbers. He was puzzled by numbers of the type $2^n - 1$, where n is a positive integer, and so he studied them further. He found that if n is composite, then $2^n - 1$ is necessarily composite. He also realised that if n is prime, $2^n - 1$ may be prime or composite. So it becomes a matter of curiosity to determine prime p for which $2^p - 1$ is a prime. Whenever a new prime is found, the probability is very high that the new prime number is of the form $2^p - 1$. As an honour to Mersenne, these numbers are called Mersenne numbers.

Mersenne asserted that the only primes between 2 and 257 for which $2^p - 1$ is prime are $p = 2, 3, 5, 7, 13, 17, 19, 31, 67, 127$ and 257. It turned out to Mersenne's misfortune, that he included one number (viz., 67) which has no place in this list and at the same time, missed one number (viz., 61) which rightfully belongs to this list—$2^{67} - 1$ is not a prime, while $2^{61} - 1$ is.

That $2^{67} - 1$ is not a prime was proved later in 1876 by Edouard Lucas (1842–1891) using the non-constructive existence proof. By this method we prove the statement indirectly without obtaining any factors explicitly.

The story of how the explicit factors of $2^{67} - 1$ were found makes for an exciting read. It was the year 1903 and the occasion was a meeting of the American Mathematical Society. At such meetings, mathematicians normally express their views by talking; they present the results of their research by lecturing. But on this occasion it was, surprisingly, a totally silent presentation of a mathematical result. The person who presented his work was Frank Nelson Cole, a professor of Columbia University, USA. The title of his paper was "On the factoring of large numbers". When his turn came, he walked silently to the board, multiplied 2 by itself 66 times, subtracted 1 from the final product and obtained the big number $147, 573, 952, 589, 676, 412, 927$. The audience was perplexed by this wordless presentation and wondered what was in the mind of the presenter Cole. They watched as Cole wrote $193, 707, 721 \times 761, 838, 257, 287$ on the board. He calculated this product, again in silence, to get the result, none other than $147, 573, 952, 589, 676, 412, 927$. After this Cole walked back to his seat gracefully but silently. The audience was speechless, but realised in an instant that what was before them were explicit big factors of the Mersenne number $2^{67} - 1$, proving constructively that it was not a prime. As soon as this dawned on the audience, they gave him a standing ovation and unrestricted applause. Cole was naturally happy to be appreciated by such an expert audience as he disclosed that he had been working on these calculations for the previous two decades. We should not forget that it was 1903, an era far removed from the calculators and computers of the present generation and so Cole's presentation well deserved the recognition it earned.

In passing, we would like to mention that Euclid had proven that if $2^n - 1$ is a prime, then $2^{(n-1)}(2^n - 1)$ is an even perfect number (defined in Lecture 5, Section 5.17). (A positive integer is called a perfect number if all its aliquote divisors i.e., all divisors except the number itself, add up to that integer, famous examples being 6, 28 etc. since $6 = 1 + 2 + 3$, and $28 = 1 + 2 + 4 + 7 + 14$).

10.13 Characterisation of Primes of the Form $4k+1$ and $4k+3$

All whole numbers $\{0, 1, 2, \ldots\}$ can be grouped into 4 categories (Table 10.1). Let k be a non-negative number.

Out of these, numbers of the form $4k$ and $4k + 2$ are clearly even (i.e., multiples of 2) and hence not primes with the sole exception of 2.

Numbers of the form $4k + 1$ and $4k + 3$ are all odd—some of them are primes and other composites. The primes in these categories behave in mutually exclusive ways as pointed out by the following two theorems incorporating their properties. These two theorems dichotomise the primes.

They were given, in 1640, by Fermat in a letter to Mersenne.

Table 10.1 Categories of whole numbers

Sl. No.	Number	Form of numbers	Description of each number in the category	Remainder that each number leaves when divided by 4
i.	{0,4,8,12,. . .}	$4k$	Exact multiple of 4	0
ii.	{1,5,9,13,. . .}	$4k + 1$	One more than a multiple of 4	1
iii.	{2,6,10,14,. . .}	$4k + 2$	Two more than a multiple of 4	2
iv.	{3,7,11,15,. . .}	$4k + 3$	Three more than a multiple of 4	3

THEOREM 1: Any number of the form (and hence any odd prime of the form) $4k + 3$ cannot be expressed as a sum $a^2 + b^2$ of two perfect squares.

THEOREM 2: The primes of the form $4k + 1$ can be expressed uniquely as the sum of two perfect squares. (NOTE: Fermat actually wrote this in geometric fashion as "A prime number which exceeds a multiple of 4 by unity is only once the hypotenuse of a right triangle)"

REMARK: It is well-known in mathematics that a converse is not necessarily true. This is observed in case of both the above theorems. We illustrate this aspect with examples:

a. Theorem 1 above states that an odd number of the form $4k + 3$ cannot be expressed as a sum of two perfect squares. This does not mean that if a number cannot be expressed as a sum of two perfect squares, it will be an odd number of the form $4k + 3$. It could be that such a number (which cannot be expressed as a sum of two perfect squares) may be even, or odd of the form $4k + 1$. For example, $12\ (= 11 + 1 = 10 + 2 = 9 + 3 = 8 + 4 = 7 + 5 = 6 + 6)$ cannot be expressed as a sum of two perfect squares, yet it is even. Similarly, $9(= 8 + 1 = 7 + 2 = 6 + 3 = 5 + 4)$ cannot be expressed as a sum of two perfect squares, but it is odd of the form $4k + 1$.

b. Theorem 2 states that a prime of the form $4k + 1$ can be expressed as a sum of two perfect squares in one and only one way. Again this does not mean that if an integer can be expressed as the sum of two perfect squares, uniquely, then it will be a prime of the form $4k + 1$ (i.e., odd prime of the form $4k + 1$). It could be that such a number will be of the form $4k + 1$(i.e., odd), but not a prime or an even and non-prime. (It could be an odd number of the form $4k + 3$ and not a prime in view of the contra-positive of Theorem 1 above). For example, $25(= 24 + 1 = 23 + 2 = 22 + 3 = 21 + 4 = 20 + 5 = 19 + 6 = 18 + 7 = 17 + 8 = 16 + 9 = 15 + 10 = 14 + 11 = 13 + 12)$ can be expressed as the sum of two perfect squares in only one way, viz, $4^2 + 3^2$, and it is of the form $4k + 1(= 4 \times 6 + 1)$, but it is not a prime. Similarly, $10(= 9 + 1 = 8 + 2 = 7 + 3 = 6 + 4 = 5 + 5)$ can be expressed as the sum of two perfect squares uniquely, viz., $3^2 + 1^2$, but it is even and non-prime.

10.14 Use of Fermat's Second Theorem to Decide Non-Primality

As pointed out by Gauss (Section 10.1), to decide whether a given number is a prime or composite is an important and useful exercise. There are different methods available to decide the primality of a given number, one of them being the sieve method taught in schools. We shall see here how Theorem 2 in Section 10.13 is useful for this purpose.

The contra-positive of Theorem 2 is: if a number of the form $4k+1$ cannot be expressed uniquely as the sum of two perfect squares, then that number is not a prime. We must clearly understand what "number cannot be expressed uniquely as the sum of two perfect squares" means. It means that the number may be expressed as the sum of two perfect squares in more than one way or it can also mean that the number cannot be expressed as the sum of two perfect squares even in one way. In both these situations, the number of the form $4k+1$ under consideration turns out not to be prime. We illustrate this now with examples.

The number 65 is of the form $4k+1(=4\times 16+1)$. It can be written as the sum of two perfect squares in two ways, namely, $65=64+1=8^2+1^2$, and $65=49+16=7^2+4^2$. Therefore by the contra-positive of Theorem 2, 65 is not a prime. In fact $65=13\times 5$.

Similarly, the number 481 is of the form $4k+1(=4\times 120+1)$. It can be written as the sum of two perfect squares in two ways, namely, $481=400+81=20^2+9^2$, and $481=225+256=15^2+16^2$. Hence by the contra-positive of Theorem 2, 481 is not a prime. In fact $481=37\times 13$.

Examples of the situation where the number cannot be expressed as the sum of two perfect squares even in one way are given below. The numbers $9(=8+1=7+2=6+3=5+4), 57(=49+8=36+21=25+32=16+41=9+48=4+53=1+56), 33(=25+8=16+17=9+24=4+29=1+32)$ are such that each of them is of the form $4k+1$, but none of them can be written as the sum of the two perfect squares. Hence by the contra-positive of Theorem 2 each of them is a composite (i.e., not prime).

Our proofs in each of the examples given above, using Theorem 2 (in fact its contra-positive) to declare that a given number was not prime, are non-constructive. We just showed that the given number although of the form $4k+1$, was not expressible uniquely as the sum of the two perfect squares, and this was sufficient to declare non-primality of the number under consideration. We did not have to give the factors of the given number explicitly. That is why the method is called non-constructive.

Incidentally, some examples of primes of the form $4k+1$ and their unique representations as the sum of two perfect squares are $61=6^2+5^2, 53=7^2+2^2, 37=1^2+6^2$.

10.15 Fermat's Factorisation Method for Deciding Primality

Gauss also said (Section 10.1) that finding factors of composite numbers is an important and useful problem. We have already discussed a non-constructive method to decide non-primality of odd integers of the form $4k+1$. Even integers are easy to recognise, as they end in 0, 2, 4, 6, or 8. They are not primes with the exception of 2. Now we give Fermat's marvellous method of factorising odd integers of any form to see whether they are primes or not. Suppose n is the odd positive integer under consideration.

STEP 1: Find m, the smallest integer $\geq \sqrt{n}$.

STEP 2: Consider the sequence of numbers $m^2 - n, (m+1)^2 - n, (m+2)^2 - n, \ldots$ and locate the smallest among them which is a perfect square. Call it q^2. So we have $p^2 - n = q^2, p^2$ being $(m+i)^2$ for the smallest i in the above sequence.

STEP 3: $n = p^2 - q^2 = (q+p)(p-q)$ giving factors of n. If the factors are 1 and n, then n is prime. Otherwise n is composite and we have its factors.

We illustrate Fermat's procedure with an example of every type.

i. $n = 75(4k+3 \text{ type})$

$\sqrt{n} \simeq 8$

$\therefore m = 9$

Now $9^2 - 75 = 6$, not a perfect square,

$10^2 - 75 = 25$, a perfect square.

$\therefore 75 = 10^2 - 5^2 = (10+5)(10-5) = 15 \times 5.$

$\therefore$ 75 is composite with factors 15 and 5.

ii. $n = 105(4k+1 \text{ type})$

$\sqrt{n} \simeq 10$

$\therefore m = 11$

Now $11^2 - 105 = 16$, a perfect square.

$\therefore 105 = 11^2 - 16 = (11+4)(11-4) = 15 \times 7.$

$\therefore$ 105 is a composite with factors 15 and 7.

iii. $n = 11(4k+3 \text{ type})$

$\sqrt{11} \simeq 3$

$\therefore m = 4$

Now $4^2 - 11 = 5$, not a perfect square.

$5^2 - 11 = 14$, not a perfect square.

$6^2 - 11 = 25$, a perfect square.

$\therefore 11 = 6^2 - 25 = (6+5)(6-5) = 11 \times 1$

$\therefore$ 11 is a prime.

iv. $n = 17(4k+1 \text{ type})$.

$\sqrt{17} \simeq 4$

$\therefore m = 5$

Now $5^2 - 17 = 8, 6^2 - 17 = 19, 7^2 - 17 = 32, 8^2 - 17 = 47,$

$9^2 - 17 = 64$, a perfect square.

$\therefore 17 = 9^2 - 64 = (9+8)(9-8) = 17 \times 1.$

$\therefore$ 17 is a prime.

10.16 Progressions with Primes

When we examine primes, we notice that the consecutive primes 3, 5, 7 form an arithmetic progression of 3 terms with a common difference of 2. Another example of a 3-term arithmetic progression of consecutive primes is 47, 53, 59, the common difference being 6. It was proved in 1944 that their exist infinitely many 3-term arithmetic progressions whose terms are primes. One such progression is 3, 7, 11. The primes 199, 409, 619, 829, 1039, 1249, 1459, 1669, 1879, and 2089 provide an example of an arithmetic progression of 10 primes with a common difference of 210. Paul Pritchard from Cornell exhibited in 1983, a 19-term arithmetic progression of primes; the first term is 8, 297, 644, 387, and the common difference is 4, 180, 566, 390.

The consecutive primes 1741, 1747, 1753, and 1759 constitute a 4-term arithmetic progression with a common difference of 6. There is a conjecture that there exist arbitrarily long arithmetic progressions of consecutive primes. This conjecture has not been proved – not even the weaker conjecture about such progressions in which the restriction that the primes be consecutive is removed.

10.17 Recent Contributions from India

With visionary insight, Gauss has underlined the significance of the problem of determining the primality of a given integer. What is required is a deterministic polynomial-time algorithm. A parallel could be the polynomial-time algorithms given by Khachian and Karmarkar for the linear programming problem in 1979 and 1984 respectively. Such an algorithm for primes had eluded the best mathematicians for several decades. Finally Manindra Agrawal (at the age of 36), a professor from IIT Kanpur, along with his two B Tech students, Neeraj Kayal (22), and Nitin Saxena (21) solved this age-old problem of finding a polynomial-time algorithm that decides whether a given number is prime or not, on August 6, 2000 – the day on which the algorithm was pasted on the IIT K website.

Conclusions

Primes and composites constitute a mine of beautiful interesting, and useful behaviour patterns. This is a vast area which has fascinated and still continues to fascinate many stalwarts. Readers will find it very fulfulling to pursue – with enthusiasm and vigour – research in this field of mathematics and collect more and more patterns of these numbers. Additional reading of [1, 7, 9] will be handy for such an endeavour.

Lecture 11

The Story of the Multi-Storey Number System

Abstract

The present lecture brings out a method of presenting numbers in a multi-storey form. The method is explained. In some cases this type of repesentation is advantageous. As an application, a "calender problem" is given.

11.1 Introduction

We all know the decimal number system. It is considered to be most appropriate and convenient in mathematical problems as well as in real-life situations. For example, the number $1\frac{1}{2}$ can be written as 1.5. It can also be written as $1.4999\ldots$ Here the digit 9 is repeated infinitely. Similarly, numbers like $\sqrt{2}$ and $\sqrt{3}$ can be expressed in decimal forms involving infinite integers after the decimal point. If we terminate the number anywhere after the decimal point, we get an approximate value.

It has been observed that some of the fine qualities of a real number system can be best understood and revealed through another presentation, namely the "multi-storey number system". It is briefly introduced below.

Consider the number $\frac{67}{29}$. We know that $2 < \frac{67}{29} < 3$.

Hence $\frac{67}{29} = 2 + x$, where x is a proper fraction. Hence

$$\frac{67}{29} = 2 + \frac{9}{29} = 2 + \cfrac{1}{\cfrac{29}{9}} = 2 + \cfrac{1}{3 + \cfrac{2}{9}}$$

$$= 2 + \cfrac{1}{3 + \cfrac{1}{\cfrac{9}{2}}} = 2 + \cfrac{1}{3 + \cfrac{1}{4 + \cfrac{1}{2}}}.$$

The number $\frac{67}{29}$ is expressed here by a 3-storey structure.

11.2 Generalisation

The method of constructing numbers in the multi-storey form should be clear from the above example. Take any number $(p/q)(q \neq 0)$, where p and q are natural numbers and follow the technique given in the illustration above. It is an easy exercise to construct multi-storey representations.

Let us generalise this idea. Consider the n-storeyed expression

$$a_0 + \cfrac{1}{a_1 + \cfrac{1}{a_2 + \ddots . a_{n-1} + \cfrac{1}{a_n}}}$$

where a_0 is a non-negative integer, $a_1, \ldots, a_n$ are natural numbers. This representation of a number is called a continued fraction and $a_0, a_1, \ldots, a_n$ are called the terms.

It is clear from the above statement that for some complicated numbers, the representation may need a full-scape paper or even a larger one. Now, is there a convenient way to represent continued fractions ? The answer to this question is, affirmative. Write

$$a_0 + \cfrac{1}{a_1 + \cfrac{1}{a_3 + \ddots . a_{n-1} + \cfrac{1}{a_n}}} = [a_0; a_1, a_2, a_3 \ldots\ldots, a_n].$$

Note the position of the semi-colon after the term a_0. Following this notation, we have,

$$\frac{67}{29} = [2; 3, 4, 2]. \text{ Further, } -\frac{67}{29} = -[2; 3.4.2].$$

Also note that

$$-\frac{67}{29} = -3 + \frac{20}{29} = -3 + \cfrac{1}{\cfrac{29}{20}} = -3 + \cfrac{1}{1 + \cfrac{9}{20}} = \ldots$$

$$= [-3; 1, 2, 4, 2].$$

Thus there are two representations to the number $-67/29$. But note that this fact does not contradict the mathematics of continued fractions.

Similarly, as an exercise, find the continued fraction for $e \approx 2.7182818284$. Naturally, our next curiosity will be: how about numbers like $\sqrt{2}, \sqrt{3}, \sqrt[3]{5}, \sqrt[4]{69}, \ldots$? These are irrational numbers. Let us take the case of $\sqrt{2}$.

Clearly $1 < \sqrt{2} < 2$. Hence there is a number x_1 such that

$$\sqrt{2} = 1 + \frac{1}{x_1}; (x_1 > 1).$$

Hence

$$\begin{aligned} x_1 &= \frac{1}{\sqrt{2}-1} = \frac{\sqrt{2}+1}{(\sqrt{2}-1)(\sqrt{2}+1)} = \sqrt{2}+1 \\ &= (1 + \frac{1}{x_1}) + 1 = 2 + \frac{1}{x_1}. \end{aligned}$$

Hence

$$\sqrt{2} = 1 + \cfrac{1}{2 + \cfrac{1}{x_1}} = 1 + \cfrac{1}{2 + \cfrac{1}{2 + \cfrac{1}{x_1}}} = 1 + \cfrac{1}{2 + \cfrac{1}{2 + \cfrac{1}{2 + \cfrac{1}{2 + \cfrac{1}{x_{1\ldots}}}}}}$$

$$= [1; 2, 2, \ldots].$$

Here the number 2 occurs infinitely. Hence it is a non-terminating continued fraction. The equality sign has been used to express $\sqrt{2}$, although it is a non-terminating continued fraction. Assume that this statement is mathematically meaningful. Let us observe such continued fractions a little closely. We have

$$x = a_0 + \cfrac{1}{a_1 + \cfrac{1}{a_2 + \ddots}} = [a_0; a_1, a_2, \ldots].$$

Then

$$\frac{1}{x} = \cfrac{1}{a_0 + \cfrac{1}{a_1 + \cfrac{1}{a_2 + \ddots}}} = [0; a_0, a_1, a_2, \ldots].$$

Following the above statement, we have

$$\frac{1}{\sqrt{2}} = [0; 1, 2, 2 \ldots].$$

Let us determine the number expressed by the non-terminating continued fraction $[0; 1, 1, \ldots]$.

Let $x = [0; 1; 1; 1; \ldots] = \cfrac{1}{1 + \cfrac{1}{1 + \cfrac{1}{1+ \ddots}}}$.

Then $\frac{1}{x} = [1; 1, 1, \ldots] = 1 + \cfrac{1}{1 + \cfrac{1}{1+ \ddots}} = 1 + x.$

Hence x satisfies the relation $x^2 + x - 1 = 0$. This is a quadratic equation. It can be solved by the standard method. Hence

$$x = \frac{-1 + \sqrt{5}}{2} \text{ or } x = \frac{-1 - \sqrt{5}}{2},$$

The second value of x is negative and is to be rejected since all terms of the given continued fraction are positive. Hence, the non-terminating continued fraction $[0; 1, 1, \ldots]$ is the number:

$$\frac{\sqrt{5} - 1}{2}.$$

This number is important in mathematical literature. It is called the "golden ratio".

The above example intuitively leads us to believe that every non-terminating continued fraction of the form $[0; a, a, \ldots]$ will end up in a quadratic equation which can be solved and that one of its roots represents the continued fraction. Is it not an interesting achievement? The generalisation of a mathematical statement enriches our intellectual experience. It then provides further insight and leads us to the detailed analysis of the theory of continued fractions.

11.3 Convergents

Now, let us consider the continued fraction $[a_0; a_1, a_2, \ldots]$.

Define $\frac{p_0}{q_0} = [a_0], \; \frac{p_1}{q_1} = [a_0; a_1], \; \frac{p_2}{q_2} = [a_0; a_1, a_2], \ldots,$

$$\frac{p_n}{q_n} = [a_0; a_1, a_2, a_3, \ldots, a_n]; n = 1, 2, 3, \ldots.$$

The numbers $(p_0/q_0), (p_1/q_1), \ldots, (p_n/q_n) \ldots$, are called the consecutive convergents of orders zero, one, ..., n respectively. For example,

$$\frac{67}{29} = [2; 3, 4, 2].$$

Here

$$\frac{p_0}{q_0} = [2] = 2; \frac{p_1}{q_1} = [2; 3] = 2 + \frac{1}{3} = \frac{7}{3} = 2.333\ldots;$$

$$\frac{p_2}{q_2} = [2; 3, 4] = \frac{30}{13} = 2.3076\ldots;$$

and

$$\frac{p_3}{q_3} = [2; 3, 4, 2] = \frac{67}{29} = 2.3103.$$

Here the convergent (p_0/q_0) is a rough approximation on the lower side of the given number (67/29), while (p_2/q_2) is a better approximation again on the lower side.

Note that (p_1/q_1) is an approximation on the upper side to the given number, while (p_3/q_3) is the actual number. A general rule which emerges out of these considerations is as follows:

Each odd-numbered convergent is greater than the neighbouring convergent, while each even-numbered convergent is less than its neighbouring convergent. Geometrically, if we plot the order of the convergent against the value of the convergent, we get the following type of graph:

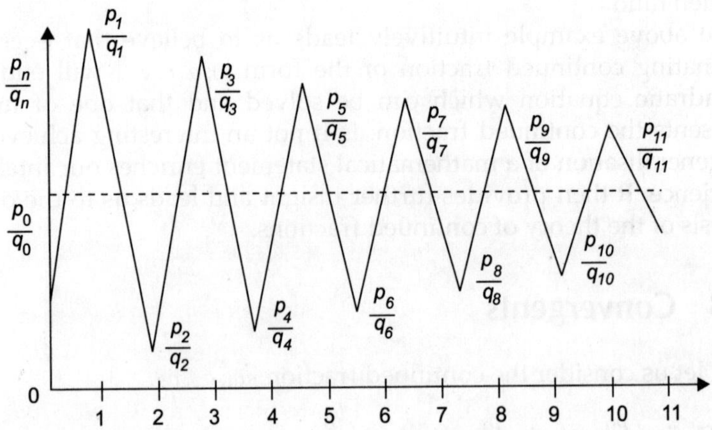

The diagram shows that the pitch of the graph goes on falling in relation to a line parallel to the order axis, indicating that (p_n/q_n), as n increases, tends to a point on the dotted line. All the odd-indexed convergents are above the dotted line, while all the even-indexed convergents are below the dotted line.

The reader should try the following exercises. Show that

$$\sqrt{3} = [1; 2, 1, 2, 1, \ldots];$$

$$\sqrt{5} = [2; 4, 4, 4, \ldots].$$

Calculate the consecutive convergents and draw the graphs in each case. Find the approximate values up to seven decimal places.

[Ans. 1.7320508, 2.2360679].

The continued fraction approximating 3.14159 is given below. Here,

$$3.14159 = 3 + 0.14159 = 3 + 0\frac{14159}{100000}$$

$$= 3 + \frac{1}{\frac{100000}{14159}} = 3 + \frac{1}{7 + \frac{62646}{1000000}}$$

$$= 3 + \frac{1}{7 + \frac{1}{\frac{1000000}{62646}}} = 3 + \frac{1}{7 + \frac{1}{15 + \frac{9671}{10000}}}$$

$$= 3 + \frac{1}{7 + \frac{1}{15 + \frac{1}{\frac{10000}{9671}}}} = 3 + \frac{1}{7 + \frac{1}{15 + \frac{1}{1 + \frac{3402}{100000}}}}.$$

Proceeding further, we get, $3.14159 = (3; 7, 15, 1, 25, 1, 7, 4)$. The successive convergents are

$$\frac{3}{1}, \frac{22}{7}, \frac{333}{106}, \frac{355}{113}, \ldots.$$

The convergent (355/113)=3.1415929. The error is 0.0000029 which is sufficiently small.

A kilometre is very nearly equal to 0.62138 miles. As an exercise, verify that the fractions 5/8, 18/29, 23/37, 64/103 are successive approximations to the ratio of a kilometre to a mile.

Generally, any mathematical idea should resemble some real-life situation. This is a very general and broad statement and hence needs some elaboration. We live in this universe. To make our life on the planet smooth, we watch our surroundings and record our experiences on our mind screen. With the gift of intellectual capacity, we try to analyse and integrate our experiences. Mathematics is also a creation of the mind. Our experiences of real-life situations recorded in the mind and mathematical ideas coincide together on several occasions. Thus our experiences get a concrete shape through the more exact language of mathematics. Let us see two such applications of the mathematics introduced above.

11.4 Calendar Problem

We know that it takes one year for the planet earth to complete one round around the sun.The tropical 1 year = 365 days 5 hours 48 minutes and 46 seconds (approximately).

The estimate of 1 year in terms of the above measures is the adopted value. It is not mathematically exact. We can say that it is very close to the actual value and in this sense we assume it to be " exact " from a practical point of view. Let us convert it into a continued fraction. We have,

5 hours 48 minutes and 46 seconds = 20926 seconds;

and

1 day = 86400 seconds.

Now,

$$1\text{year} = \left(365 + \frac{20926}{86400}\right) \text{days} = \left(365 + \frac{10463}{43200}\right) \text{days}$$

$$= 365 + \frac{1}{\frac{43200}{10463}} = 365 + \frac{1}{4 + \frac{1348}{10463}} = 365 + \frac{1}{4 + \frac{1}{\frac{10463}{1348}}}$$

$$= 365 + \cfrac{1}{4 + \cfrac{1}{7 + \cfrac{1}{1 + \cfrac{1}{3 + \cfrac{1}{\frac{321}{64}}}}}} = 365 + \cfrac{1}{4 + \cfrac{1}{7 + \cfrac{1}{1 + \cfrac{1}{3 + \cfrac{1}{5 + \frac{1}{64}}}}}}$$

$$= [365; 4, 7, 1, 3, 5, 64] \text{ days.}$$

We now calculate the consecutive convergents. Below d stands for day, h for hour, m for minutes and s for seconds. We have

$$\frac{p_0}{q_0} = [365] = 365\,\text{d};$$

$$\frac{p_1}{q_1} = [365; 4] = 365\frac{1}{4}\,\text{d} = 365\,\text{d}\ 06\,\text{h}\ 00\,\text{m}\ 00\,\text{s};$$

$$\frac{p_2}{q_2} = [365; 4, 7] = 365\,\frac{7}{29}\ \text{days} = 365\,\text{d}\ 05\,\text{h}\ 47\,\text{m}\ 35\,\text{s};$$

$$\frac{p_3}{q_3} = [365; 4, 7, 1] = 365\,\frac{8}{33}\ \text{days} = 365\,\text{d}\ 05\,\text{h}\ 49\,\text{m}\ 05\,\text{s};$$

$$\frac{p_4}{q_4} = [365; 4, 7, 1, 3] = 365\,\frac{31}{128}\ \text{days} = 365\,\text{d}\ 05\,\text{h}\ 48\,\text{m}\ 45\,\text{s}.$$

We find from the convergents that $\frac{p_0}{q_0}$, $\frac{p_2}{q_2}$, $\frac{p_4}{q_4}$, are the lower approximations to the actual value assumed. The errors, in these values from the "exact" value, are

5 h 48 m 46 s 1 m 11 s, 1 s

respectively. We find that the error goes on decreasing and in fact, if we assume (p_4/q_4) as the value, then the error is just one second.

As against these, the convergents $\frac{p_1}{q_1}$, $\frac{p_3}{q_3}$ are upper approximations to the "exact" value. The errors committed are 11 m 14 s, and 19 s respectively. Here also the error goes on decreasing.

For practical purposes, our 1 year is equal to 365 days i.e., the convergent (p_0/q_0). Clearly this is a much lower estimate than the "exact" value. If we assume (p_1/q_1) as a year, then we have to account for 6 hours time each year. In four years the mistake accumulated is 24 hours. Hence to compensate for this mistake, it is a practice to add one day to every fourth year and call it a leap year. But note that in the assumption that (p_1/q_1) is equal to a year, we again commit an upward mistake of 11 m 14 s each year. In a century, the accumulated mistake is 18 h 43 m 20 s. The accumulated mistake is compensated by not considering the century year as a leap year i.e., each century year has 28 days in February. But then we commit a mistake of 24 hours − (18 h 43 m 20 s) = 5 h 16 m 40 s. In four consecutive centuries, this mistake grows to 21 h 6 m 40 s. To cover this mistake, the 4th century year is treated as a leap year. Since year 2000 is divisible by 400, it is a leap year and February of the year 2000 has 29 days.

Naturally the story does not end here since there is a mistake of 2 h 53 m 20 s in every 400 years. This mistake needs to be compensated. But since it only has to be accounted after almost 32 centuries, we can leave it to the care of a future generation of human beings. But young students should go on calculating the mistakes thus committed in thousands of years in the future. Is it not a good exercise?

From the above discussions we can see that there is an advantage in becoming a student of mathematics. From the convergents, it is naturally seen that the next convergent (p_4/q_4) is a better approximation to a year. Here the mistake is $31/128$ days every year when compared with (p_0/q_0) (convergent in vogue). The advantage is that the mistake here is only one second every year. Then from $31/128$ days every year, we find that we will need only 31 leap years in 128 years and the year 128 is to be treated as a non-leap year. But this scheme is not accepted since the numbers involved here are difficult for a lay man to calculate. When there is total mathematical literacy all over the world, people may accept (p_4/q_4) as a best estimate for the time-scale of one year.

One may assume 1 year $=$ 365.24226 days. Convert 0.24226 into a continued fraction and find the sequence of convergents. The story of multi-storey numbers appears to be continuing forever.

Conclusion

The method of continued fractions is explained and its advantages are illustrated through a real-life problem [see reference 1]. This branch of mathematics has several applications. For example, our ancient Indian mathematicians took considerable interest in a branch of mathematics named "indeterminate equations". It needs continued fractions on several occasions. This method has also applications in differential equations. The reader can prepare mathematical projects by reading the references [2,3].

Lecture 12

Festival of Triangles

Abstract

In the present lecture we aim to build a relationship between rational numbers, geometry and difference equations. The geometrical figure under consideration will be a triangle. This is a simple figure introduced in the school curriculum at an elementary level. Students are taught some properties of triangles but quite a lot remains unexplored. We will see that the properties of triangles, their families grouped according to certain conditions have been under investigation since historical times. This fact can be verified from the references which are listed at the end. It is difficult to discuss here the entire range of results obtained on triangles since time immemorial. We present only a few of them.

12.1 Introduction

Firstly, we consider the Pythagorean triangles. Associated with each triangle are numbers like the perimeter and the area of a triangle. We can obtain the ratio of these numbers and construct families of triangles having integer sides. Such triangles are also called rational triangles. Other properties like radius of the incircle, circumscribed circle, escribed circles, the trigonometrical ratios etc., have special relationships with the integer sides of a triangle. These relationships are often expressed in terms of difference equations, a topic in higher mathematics. The results are both precise and rewarding and provide enough scope for further investigations.

12.2 Pythagorean Triangles

In the study of the properties of triangles, right-angled triangles provide more fodder for the curious-minded. In particular, right-angled triangles with integer sides have been studied over several centuries. These are called "Pythagorean triangles". They are also often as denoted as "Pythagorean triplets".

In ancient India, the mathematicians Baudhayan and Apastamba have written about such triangles in the *Sulvasutras*. This dates back to the 5th century BCE or even before. They discovered that the triplets

$$\left[x, \frac{x^2-1}{2}, \frac{x^2+1}{2}\right],$$

when x is an odd number; and

$$\left[x, \frac{1}{4}x^2-1, \frac{1}{4}x^2+1\right],$$

when x is an even number, are Pythagorean.

The famous Greek mathematician Pythagoras, himself considered the triplet $(x, y, z) = (2\alpha+1, 2\alpha^2+2\alpha, 2\alpha^2+2\alpha+1)$, where α is any positive integer and proved that $x^2+y^2=z^2$.

Another great scholar, Diophantus, assumed that the triplet,

$$(x, y, z) = \left(\frac{2mz}{m^2+1}, \frac{m^2-1}{m^2+1}z, z\right),$$

where m and z are any positive integers was pythagorean. Similar relationship exists if we choose $(x, y, z) = (2mn, m^2-n^2, m^2+n^2)$ where m, n are positive integers, as a triplet. This example was given by Brahmagupta.

L Kronecker proved that all possible solutions of the equation $x^2+y^2 = z^2$ are given by $x = 2pqt, y = t(p^2-q^2)$, $z = t(p^2+q^2); p > 0, q > 0, t > 0$; p and q are relatively prime and are not both odd.

It is possible to construct more than one Pythagorean triangle with the same perimeter. For example, triangles $(24, 45, 51), (20, 48, 52), (30, 40, 50)$ are three Pythagorean triplets having the perimeter 120.

Only a few families of Pythagorean triangles have been mentioned in the above discussion. It is possible to consider Pythagorean triplets having additional merits like integral areas, integral medians, integral bisectors etc. The reader is encouraged to undertake such projects.

12.3 Perimeter–Area Relations

For each non-trivial triangle we have two associated numbers, namely, the perimeter and the area. A question can be asked if there exists some relationship between the two numbers: Can we formulate families of triangles in which there exists some relation between the perimeter and its area? In the section we will present a partial answer.

Let (a, b, c) denote the integer-valued sides of a triangle ABC. Denote by $2s = a + b + c$, the perimeter of the Δ ABC. Let A denote the area. Suppose that $2s : A = \mu : 1$, i.e. $2s = A\mu, \mu > 0$. We then can consider the possibilities: (i) $\mu < 1$, (ii) $\mu = 1$ and (iii) $\mu > 1$. In addition, we may consider some selected values for a, b, and c. Much research has been done on the perimeter–area relationship. This study still continues and provides open challenges to mathematicians by posing new problems. In fact, a triangle, is the simplest diagram in geometry, yet many of its properties still remain undiscovered. We will consider a few of such studies to indicate what has been done and what can be explored in the future.

12.3.1

In introductory textbooks of trigonometry under the section on "properties of triangles," we meet with a formula which relates the area and the perimeter of a triangle, namely,

$$A = \sqrt{s(s-a)(s-b)(s-c)}, 2s = a + b + c. \tag{1}$$

This formula was given by Heron of Alexandria. Heron showed that the triangle $(13, 14, 15)$ has area 84. A triangle with rational sides and with rational area is called a "Heron triangle". Essentially in this section we will restrict our studies to Heron triangles.

The well-known Indian mathematician, Bramhagupta (598 CE) noted that if a, b, c are any rational numbers, then

$$\frac{1}{2}\left(\frac{a^2}{b} + b\right), \frac{1}{2}\left(\frac{a^2}{c} + c\right), \frac{1}{2}\left(\frac{a^2}{b} - b\right) + \frac{1}{2}\left(\frac{a^2}{c} - c\right);$$

A triangle with these sides has its altitude and areas as rational numbers. This fact suggests that the problem under consideration has been thought of several centuries before.

A Japanese mathematician, Nakane Genkei, in the year 1722 considered triangles whose sides are consecutive integers, such that the perpendicular upon the longest side from the opposite vertex is an integer. With this restriction, he discovered the triangles $(3, 4, 5), (13, 14, 15), (51, 52, 53), (193, 194, 195)$. Let such triangles be denoted by triplets $(a_r, b_r, c_r), r = 1, 2, 3, \ldots$. Clearly $a_1 = 3, a_2 = 13, a_3 = 51, a_4 = 193, \ldots$. The first few a_is can be determined by inspection but soon the process becomes complicated. In order to find values of a_r, $r = 5, 6, 7, \ldots$, we need to exploit mathematical tools. For this purpose we use the method of difference equations. Let us consider a recurrence relation $a_{r+1} = \alpha a_r + \beta a_{r-1} + \chi$;

$r = 2, 3, 4, \ldots$. Here the coefficients α, β, χ are constants to be determined. For $r = 2$,

$$a_3 = \alpha a_2 + \beta a_1 + \chi$$

and for

$$r = 3, a_4 = \alpha a_3 + \beta a_2 + \chi.$$

Hence, we get two equations (after substituting a_1, a_2, a_3, a_4),

$$13\alpha + 3\beta + \chi = 51$$

$$51\alpha + 13\beta + \chi = 193;$$

which yield $38\alpha + 10\beta = 142$.

By inspection, we get $\alpha = 4$ and $\beta = -1$ and finally $\chi = 2$. Thus the recurrence relation is given by

$$a_{r+1} = 4a_r - a_{r-1} + 2; r = 2, 3, 4, \ldots.$$

For $r = 4$, we have

$$a_5 = 4a_4 - a_3 + 2 = 723.$$

Hence, $(a_5, b_5, c_5) = (723, 724, 725)$.

This triangle has the desired properties. From a_5, a_4, a_3, we can now construct a_6. The process continues indefinitely and we can completely determine all members of the family (a_j, b_j, c_j).

This family of triangles is infinite. The areas of the respective triangles are $6, 84, 1170, 16296, \ldots$. In fact, one can obtain recurrence relations of these numbers too by following the above method.

12.3.2

Let m be any positive integer. Consider a triangle having sides $2m^2 + 1, 2m^2 + 2, 4m^2 + 1$. Clearly, $2s = 8m^2 + 4$. Now,

$$A^2 = s(s-a)(s-b)(s-c) = (4m^2 + 2)(2m^2 + 1)(2m^2)(1)$$

$$= 4m^2(2m^2 + 1)^2.$$

Thus,

$$A = 2m(2m^2 + 1) = 1, 2, 3, \ldots,$$

We can now state the results in the following table:

m	A	**Triangle triplet**	$2s$	$\frac{2s}{A} = \mu$
1	6	(3,4,5)	12	2
2	36	(9,10,17)	36	1
3	114	(19,20,37)	76	1/3
4	264	(33,34,65)	132	1/2
5	510	(51,52,101)	204	2/5
6	876	(73,74,145)	292	1/3
⋮	⋮	⋮	⋮	⋮

This table can be extended further. Observe that here the value of μ is decreasing. Note that for $m \geq 3, \mu < 1$. Hence we conclude that for $\mu < 1$, there is an infinite family of triangles. In case $m = 1$ and $m = 2$, we have $\mu = 2$ and $\mu = 1$ respectively. We need separate consideration for such cases.

12.3.3

We consider below a triangle (a, b, c), where a, b and c are integers. First, we consider the case where $\mu = 2s/A = 1$, i.e., the perimeter of a triangle and its area are equal. It was proved by W A Whitworth and D Biddle (Refer to the book by L E Dickson, *History of the Theory of Numbers*, Vol. II. page 199) that the only five triangles possessing this property are $(9, 10, 17), (7, 15, 20), (6, 25, 29), (6, 8, 10)$ and $(5, 12, 13)$. We do not provide here the proof of this statement. The readers can verify that the area and perimeter of these triangles are equal. Constructing the proof is a challenge which can be taken up by interested readers.

Let us now consider the case where $\mu = (2s/A) = 2$, i.e., the perimeter of a rational triangle is two times the area of a triangle. By intuition, we have a rational triangle $(a, b, c) = (3, 4, 5)$ having the perimeter 12 and area $A = 6$. We wish to conclude here that this is the only triangle possessing this desired property. Thus the triangle $(3, 4, 5)$ is the only triplet which forms a perfect triangle.

Here we give a line of proof. For a rational triplet (a, b, c), $a \leq b \leq c$, we have

$$A^2 = s(s - a)(s - b)(s - c).$$

For $s = A$, we have $A = (A - a)(A - b)(A - c)$.

Let $X = A - a, Y = A - b, Z = A - c$, clearly, $x \leq y \leq z$,

so that we get $A = XYZ$ and $X + Y + Z = A$. (verify).

Hence $XYZ = X + Y + Z$.

This is a non-linear equation in X, Y, Z. We will try to get the values for X, Y and Z.

Now consider $Y(YZ-1) \leq X(YZ-1) = XYZ - X = Y + Z < 2Y$,

or $YZ - 1 < 2$.

Further, since $X \geq Y \geq Z$, we obtain $Z^2 \leq YZ \leq 3$.

Clearly, $Z = 1$ is the only integer solution of this inequality.

Hence $Y + 1 = XY - X = X(Y-1)$.

For $Y = 2$, this relation yields $X = 3$.

Hence, $(X, Y, Z) = (3, 2, 1)$, so that $(a, b, c) = (3, 4, 5)$.

The above conclusion is equivalent to saying that the curve $XY - X - Y - 1 = 0$ passes through the integer coordinate point (3, 2) and none other.

12.3.4

In the present sub-section, we continue to study the relationship between the perimeter and the area of a rational triangle. A simple rational triangle $(a, b, c) = (3, 4, 5)$ illustrates the nature of the problem to be solved. We note the following features of this triangle.

1. The sides of the triangle are consecutive integers,
2. (a, b, c) is a Pythagorean triplet,
3. $\mu = 2$ and
4. area A is an integer.

Suppose someone raises the question: Is there any other triangle satisfying the features (1–4) given above? It has been proved that $(3, 4, 5)$ is the only triangle possessing all the four features given above. However if we delete the feature (2) and (3), we can obtain a family of triangles having the features (1) and (4) and show that the family consists of infinite members. Further, we will investigate the other properties of such triangles like inscribed, circumscribed, escribed circles. For completeness, we provide some properties of triangles below:

i. Heron's formula for the area of a triangle in terms of its perimeter is given in (1),

ii. r =(Area/s) $= (s-a)\tan$ A/2. (Here A is any one angle of the triangle ABC having sides (a, b, c) and r is the radius of the inscribed circle.

iii. Let R denote the radius of the circumscribed circle, r_a, r_b, r_c denote the radii of the escribed circles related to the sides a, b, c. The following relations are known:

a. $\dfrac{1}{r} = \dfrac{1}{r_a} + \dfrac{1}{r_b} = \dfrac{1}{r_c},$

b. $r_a = \dfrac{A}{s-a}, r_b = \dfrac{A}{s-b}, r_c = \dfrac{A}{s-c},$

c. $r_a + r_b + r_c = r + 4R,$

d. $R = 2r + \dfrac{1}{2r},$

e. $R = \dfrac{abc}{4A}.$

Since the sides of a triangle are consecutive integers, let us assume that $a = u - 1, b = u$, and $c = u + 1$, where $u > 1$ is an integer, so that the perimeter $2s = 3u$, and

$$A^2 = s(s-a)(s-b)(s-c) = \frac{3u^2(u^2-4)}{16}.$$

We need A to be an integer. This means the RHS is an integer

In order to cancel 16 in the above expression, u must be an even number. Further $(u^2(u^2-4)/16))$ must be a multiple of 3. Clearly u^2 cannot be a multiple of 3 without also being a multiple of 9. Hence we conclude that, for a suitable integer ν

$$u^2 - 4 = 3\,\nu^2,$$

or

$$u^2 - 3\,\nu^2 = 4. \tag{2}$$

This is a Diophantine equation in u. We need to find a solution u which is an even integer. Equations of this kind are studied with several details in literature. This equation has the form $u^2 - D\,\nu^2 = 4, D > 0, D$ is not a square of any integer.

The method of finding solutions of such equations involves finding at least one solution (u_1, ν_1) by inspection. This solution should be a minimal solution, i.e., lowest possible positive pair (u_1, ν_1). Then the general solution is given by

$$u + \nu\sqrt{D} = 2\left(\frac{u_1 + \nu_1\sqrt{D}}{2}\right)^n, n = 1, 2, 3, \ldots.$$

In case of the equation (2), by inspection $(u_1, \nu_1) = (4, 2)$. Clearly $u_1 = 4$ and $\nu_1 = 2$ and $D = 3$. Hence the minimal solution may be taken as $4 + 2\sqrt{3}$. The general solution is then given by

$$u + \nu\sqrt{D} = u + \nu\sqrt{3} = 2\left[\frac{4 + 2\sqrt{3}}{2}\right]^n = 2\left[2 + \sqrt{3}\right]^n, n = 1, 2, 3, \ldots.$$

For each n, we have a solution, hence we write $u = u_n$ and $\nu = \nu_n$ and state the general solution in the form,

$$u_n + \nu_n\sqrt{3} = 2\left[2 + \sqrt{3}\right]^n, \; n = 1, 2, 3, \ldots. \quad (3)$$

For $n = 1$, we have $u_1 = 4$ and $\nu_1 = 2$. Hence the triplet $(u_1 - 1, u_1, u_1 + 1) = (3, 4, 5)$, a triangle with which we started.

For $n = 2$, $u_2 + \nu_2\sqrt{3} = 2\left[2 + \sqrt{3}\right]^2 = 14 + 4\sqrt{3}$. Hence $u_2 = 14$, $\nu_2 = 4$, is clearly a solution of (2). The triplet $(u_2 - 1, u_2, u_2 + 1) = (13, 14, 15)$ provides the next triangle in the family. We can now take $n = 3, 4, 5, \ldots$ and obtain successive members of the family. The following table lists the first five triangles having the desired property.

n	$u_n - 1$	u_n	$u_n + 1$	A_n **(Area)**
1	3	4	5	6
2	13	14	15	84
3	51	52	53	1170
4	193	194	195	16,296
5	723	724	725	2,28,144

Observe that for large n, u_n will be a large number. For $n = 20$, $u_n = 275758382274$. Obviously the number A_{20} will also be a large number. Although the above table contains 5 triangles, it is clear that the formula (3) provides us infinite family members

We now proceed to study the sequences $\{u_n\}$ and $\{A_n\}$. As in the subsection 12.3.1, we proceed to find the recurrence relation satisfied by u_n. Let

$$u_{n+2} + \alpha u_{n+1} + \beta u_n + \chi = 0, n = 1, 2, 3, \ldots.. \; u_1 = 4, \; u_2 = 14.$$

We then prove that $\alpha = -4, \beta = 1$ and $\chi = 0$ by using the initial data. Thus we have the recurrence relation

$$u_{n+2} = 4u_{n+1} - u_n, u_1 = 4, u_2 = 14, \; n = 2, 3, 4, \ldots.. \quad (4)$$

The theory of difference equations, gives rise to many methods to solve equations of this type. The characteristic equation for the above difference equation is given by $r^2 - 4r + 1 = 0$ having roots $2 \pm \sqrt{3}$. Hence the solutions of the difference equations (4) are given by

$$u_n = [2+\sqrt{3}]^n + [2-\sqrt{3}]^n, n = 1, 2, 3, \ldots.$$

We have clearly obtained the values of u_1 to u_5 in the given table. The difference equation or the solution given above helps us to build up the family members for $n = 6, 7, 8, \ldots$

Further, note that the first few elements of the sequence $\{A_n\}$, given in the above table, suggests that there exists a recurrence relation in this sequence. We can obtain this recurrence relation in $\{A_n\}$ by following the known technique. It is given by

$$A_{n+2} = 14\ A_{n+1} - A_n\ ; n = 2, 3, 4, \ldots \tag{5}$$

To find the expression for its solution, note that the characteristic equation of (5) is

$r^2 - 14r + 1 = 0$ having roots $7 \pm 4\sqrt{3}$. Hence,

$$A_n = \frac{\sqrt{3}}{4}\left\{(7+4\sqrt{3})^n - (7-4\sqrt{3})^n\right\}.$$

$$= \frac{\sqrt{3}}{4}\left\{(2+\sqrt{3})^{2n} - (2-\sqrt{3})^{2n}\right\}, n = 2, 3, 4, \ldots.$$

Further, it is possible to connect the elements of the sequences $\{u_n\}$ and $\{A_n\}$. From the earlier expression for u_n, observe that

$$16A_n^2 = 3u_n^2(u_n^2 - 4).$$

Further $u_n^2 = [(2+\sqrt{3})^n + (2-\sqrt{3})^n]^2$

$$= \left[(2-\sqrt{3})^{2n} + (2-\sqrt{3})^{2n} + 2\right] = u_{2n} + 2.$$

Now $\quad 16A_n^2 = 3u_n^2(u_n^2 - 4)$

$$= 3(u_{2n} + 2)(u_{2n} - 2)$$

$$= 3(u_{2n}^2 - 4);$$

i.e., $A_n^2 = \dfrac{3}{16}(u_{2n}^2 - 4) = \dfrac{3}{16}(u_{4n} - 2).$

Now, we turn our attention to finding the radii r of incircles of this family of triangles.

We have, $\quad r_n^2 = \dfrac{A_n^2}{s_n^2}, \quad n = 1, 2, 3, \ldots$

$$= \frac{3u_n^2(u_n^2-4)}{16.\left(\frac{3u_n}{2}\right)^2} = \frac{u_n^2-4}{12}$$

$$= \frac{u_{2n}-2}{12}$$

For $\quad n = 1, r_1^2 = \frac{u_2-2}{12} = \frac{14-2}{12} = 1$, i.e., $r_1 = 1$,

and when $n = 2, r_2^2 = \frac{u_4-2}{12} = \frac{194-2}{12} = 16, r_2 = 4.$

We obtain r for $n = 3, 4, 5, \ldots$, and formulate the sequence $\{r_n\}$ of incircles' radii. Here

$$\{r_n\} = \{1, 4, 15, 56, 209, 780, 2911, 10864, \ldots\}.$$

The elements of this sequence satisfy the recurrence relation

$$r_{n+2} = 4r_{n+1} - r_n.\ n = 2, 3, 4, \ldots.$$

Let us now try to find the radii of the escribed circles, given by

$$r_a = \frac{rs}{s-a}, r_b = \frac{rs}{s-b}, r_c = \frac{rs}{s-c},$$

where r is the radius of the incircle.

Clearly, $(r_n)_a^2 = \frac{r_n^2 s_n^2}{(s_n-a)^2}$

$$= \frac{\frac{u_n^2-4}{12}.\left(\frac{3u_n}{2}\right)^2}{\left(\frac{3u_n}{2}-(u_n-1)\right)^2} = \frac{1}{4}u_n^2\left(\frac{u_n^2+2}{u_n^2-2}\right).$$

Here $(r_n)_a$ denotes the radius of the escribed circle opposite to the angle A of Δ ABC. This relation gives the square of the radius of the escribed circle related to the side a i.e., u_{n-1}. Similarly,

$(r_n)_b^2 = \frac{3}{4}(u_n^2 - 4)$ related to the side $b = u_n$ and

$(r_n)_c^2 = \frac{3}{4}u_n^2\,(u_n - 2/u_n + 2)$ related to the side $c = u_{n+1}$.

Observe that $r_n, (r_n)_a, (r_n)_b, (r_n)_c$ are all rational numbers. The consequent sequences are given by

$$\{r_n\}_a = \left\{6.14, \frac{234}{5}, \frac{679}{4}, \frac{11946}{19}, \ldots\right\}$$

$$\{r_n\}_b = \{3.12, 48, 168, 2340, \ldots\}$$

$$\{r_n\}_c = \left\{2, \frac{21}{2}, \frac{130}{3}, \frac{1164}{7}, \frac{6878}{11}, \frac{50795}{13} \ldots\right\}, n = 1, 2, 3 \ldots..$$

To check the relation

$$\frac{1}{r} = \frac{1}{r_a} + \frac{1}{r_b} + \frac{1}{r_c}, \text{ for } n = 1,$$

we have $r = 1, r_a = 6, r_b = 3, r_c = 2$, and hence the relation holds.

The other relations may be verified. In addition to noting that $(r_n)_a, (r_n)_b, (r_n)_c$ are rational numbers, the sequence $(r_n)_b$ is that of integers.

In particular, consider the triplet $(13, 14, 15)$ of the family of triangles having area 84. One of the radii of the escribed circle is 12. It is noted here that the escribed radius 12 and sides of the triangle 13, 14, 15 are consecutive numbers. In fact, it is known that one of the altitudes of this triangle is again 12. This is the only triangle in the family possessing such striking properties.

We have yet to consider the radius of the circumcircle of a triangle belonging to this family. It is known that $R = (abc/4A)$. For n, we have

$$R_n = \frac{a_n b_n c_n}{4A_n}$$

$$R_n^2 = \frac{[(u_n - 1)(u_n)(u_n + 1)]^2}{16A_n^2}$$

$$= \frac{u_n^2(u_n^2 - 1)}{16\dfrac{3u_n^2(u_n^2 - 4)}{16}} \text{ (substituting } A_n)$$

$$= \frac{\frac{1}{3}(u_n^2 - 1)^2}{u_n^2 - 4}; n = 1, 2, 3 \ldots$$

This relation helps us to construct the sequence $\{R_n\}$ and is given by

$$\{R_n\} = \{5/2, 65/8, 901/30, 12545/112, 174725/418, \ldots\},$$

We can now check that $R_1 = 2r_1 + (1/2r_1)$, where $r_1 = 1.[r_1$ is the radius of the incircle of the triangle triplet $(3, 4, 5)]$. Clearly, $R_1 = 5/2$, the first element of the above sequence.

We now turn to some trigonometric properties of triangles belonging to this family. From properties of triangles we know that

$$2 \text{ Area} = ab \sin \text{C} = bc \sin \text{A} = ca \sin \text{B}.$$

Substitute for A, a, b, c for each value of n to get

$$\sin^2 A_n = \left[\frac{2\text{ area}}{b_n c_n}\right]^2$$

$$= \frac{4(\text{area})^2}{b_n^2\, c_n^2} = \frac{4.3u_n^2(u_n^2-4)}{16.u_n^2(u_n+1)^2} = \frac{3}{4}\frac{u_n^2-4}{(u_n+1)^2}.$$

Similarly

$$\sin^2 B_n = \frac{3}{4}\frac{u_n^2(u_n^2-4)}{(u_n^2-1)^2};$$

and

$$\sin^2 C_n = \frac{3}{4}\frac{u_n^2-4}{(u_n^2-1)^2}$$

Here A_n, B_n, C_n represent angles of the nth triangle of the family.

Clearly all sine ratios of the angles of all triangles in the family are rational numbers. Now, let $n \to \infty$, then $\sin^2 A_n, \sin^2 B_n, \sin^2 C_n$ all tend to 3/4 i.e., for large n

$$(\sin A_n, \sin B_n, \sin C_n) \approx \left(\frac{\sqrt{3}}{2}, \frac{\sqrt{3}}{2}, \frac{\sqrt{3}}{2}\right)$$

This is a case of an equilateral triangle. For large integers n, the three consecutive numbers $(u_n - 1, u_n, u_n + 1)$ almost form an equilateral triangle.

So far, we have obtained a few properties of triangles belonging to the family. Study of this kind can proceed further. For example, a triangle has medians, altitudes, orthocentre, incentre, centroid, nine-point circle, centres of escribed circles. All these lines and points are related to each other by several geometrical properties. One can study such a geometry for infinite members of this family of triangles. Relations established so far are sufficient to proceed further.

In the above family, we assumed that the sides are consecutive integers. This assumption may be replaced by taking the sides as $2u-1, u, 2u+1$, where $u \geq 2$ is an integer. Let us study the triangles for integral areas. Here

$$s = 5u/2, s-a = \frac{u+2}{2}, s-b = \frac{3u}{2}, s-c = \frac{u-2}{2} \text{ and}$$

$$A^2 = s(s-a)(s-b)(s-c) = 15u^2(u^2-4)/16;$$

an expression similar to the one we obtained at the beginning of this sub-section. Arguing on similar lines we have a Diophantine equation,

$$u^2 - 15\nu^2 = 4;$$

having the minimal solution $u_1 = 8, \nu_1 = 2$.

Now for $u_1 = 8, \nu_1 = 2$, we have $A_1 = 60$. Following a similar procedure given in the earlier discussion, we establish a family of triangles. Here the first triangle

$$(2u_1 - 1, u_1, 2u_1 + 1) = (15, 8, 17).$$

The other triangles, areas and trigonometrical ratios can be obtained similarly. The details are omitted.

12.3.5

The discussion of the present problem leads to a generalisation in which we consider a rational triangle having sides $n - r, n, n + r$ (when $r = 1$, the triangle under consideration has sides $n - 1, n, n + 1$ which are three consecutive numbers, thus covering the earlier situation).

For the triangle $(n - r, n, n + r)$, $2s = 3n$ and

$$A^2 = s(s - a)(s - b)(s - c) = \frac{3n^2}{16}(n^2 - 4r^2).$$

We have to find n and r such that A is an integer. We again end the discussion here and leave the calculations to the reader.

12.4 A Converse Problem for Rational Triangles

In the earlier section, we considered the rational triplet (a, b, c) and attempted to find the number of triangles under various restrictions. The converse problem is: given the rational perimeter $2s$, how many rational triangles (a, b, c) can be obtained? This fact amounts to asking " how many rational partitions of integer $2s$, in triplets, are possible so that viable rational triangles can be formed?" Observe that for a given integer, there may exist triplet partitions but each partition may not form a triangle. We know that for a triangle to be formed, a " triangle inequality" needs to be satisfied. In mathematical terms, our a, b, c should be such that

i. $a + b + c = n$ (n is a pre-assigned positive integer)

ii. the sum of any two of a, b, c is greater than the third number.

We aim to determine the number of triplets (a, b, c) satisfying the conditions (i) and (ii) above. Let T_n donote this number.

When the given number n is small, we can obtain T_n by inspection. For large numbers, this method fails. We list below n, (a, b, c) and T_n for some simple situations.

n	(a, b, c)	T_n	Remark
1	$(1, 0, 0)$	0	Trivial triangle
2	$(1, 1, 0)$	0	Trivial triangle
3	$(1, 1, 1)$	1	
4	$(1, 1, 2)$ $(2, 2, 0)$	0	Both are trivial triangles
5	$(2, 2, 1)$	1	
6	$(2, 2, 2)$	1	
7	$(3, 2, 2)$ $(3, 3, 1)$	2	
8	$(3, 3, 2)$	1	
9	$(3, 3, 3)$ $(3, 4, 2)$ $(4, 4, 1)$	3	
10	$(4, 4, 2)$ $(3, 4, 3)$	2	
11	$(5, 4, 2)$ $(5, 3, 3)$ $(4, 4, 3)(5, 5, 1)$	4	
12	$(4, 4, 4)$ $(5, 5, 2)$ $(5, 4, 3)$	3	
13	$(6, 6, 1)$ $(6, 5, 2)$ $(6, 4, 3)$ $(5, 5, 3)$ $(5, 4, 4)$	5	
14	$(6, 6, 2)$ $(6, 5, 3)$ $(6, 4, 4)$ $(5, 5, 4)$	4	

NOTE: For $n = 7$, we have (7, 0, 0), (6, 1, 0), (5, 2, 0), (5, 1, 1), (4, 3, 0), (4, 2, 1), (3, 2, 2), (3, 3, 1) partitions but only the last two triplets form non-trivial triangles. The above table takes into account the number of non-trivial triangles T_n only.

The following result is known. We state it here without proof.

Let a, b, c be the integer sides of a triangle having perimeter n. Assume without loss of generality that $a \geq b \geq c$. The number T_n satisfies the following relation

$$T_n = \begin{cases} T_{n-3} & \text{when } n \text{ is even;} \\ T_{n-3} + \dfrac{n}{4} + \dfrac{(-1)^{\frac{n+1}{2}}}{4} & \text{when } n \text{ is odd.} \end{cases}$$

We can easily verify this relation for $n = 4, 6, 8, 10, 12, 14$ and for $n = 3, 5, 7, 9, 11, 13$ and verify the above table. For example,

$$T_{13} = T_{10} + \frac{13}{4} + \frac{(-1)^{14/2}}{4}$$

$$= 2 + 3 + \frac{1}{4} - \frac{1}{4} = 5$$

With the help of this result we can build up the above table further.

It was discovered that if we expand the expression

$$\frac{x^3}{(1-x^2)(1-x^3)(1-x^4)} = x^3(1-x^2)^{-1}(1-x^3)^{-1}(1-x^4)^{-1}$$

into a power series and consider the coefficients of powers of x, we get the sequence $1, 0, 1, 1, 2, 1, 3, 2, 4, \ldots$ which is the sequence $T_3, T_4, \ldots, T_{11}$ given in the table. This sequence of numbers is called " Alcuin's sequence ". It is found that the given expression is a generating function for T_n. Suppose that $T(x)$ is the generating function given by the infinite series,

$$T(x) = T_0 + T_1 x + T_2 x^2 + \ldots$$

then

$$x^3 T(x) = T_0 x^3 + T_1 x^4 + T_2 x^5 + T_3 x^6 + T_4 x^7 + \ldots.$$

Hence

$$(1-x^3)T(x) = T_0 + T_1 x + T_2 x^2 + (T_3 - T_0)x^3 + (T_4 - T_1)x^4 + (T_5 - T_2)x^5 + \ldots.$$

Here from the table $T_0 = T_1 = T_2 = 0$. Hence, using the table for T_n further,

$$(1-x^3)T(x) = x^3 + x^5 + 2x^7 + 2x^9 + 3x^{11} + 3x^{13} + \ldots$$

$$= x^3(1+x^2).(1+2x^4+3x^8+\ldots)$$

$$= x^3(1+x^2(1-x^4)^{-2})$$

$$= \frac{x^3(1+x^2)}{(1-x^4)^2}$$

Hence

$$T(x) = \frac{x^3(1+x^2)}{(1-x^3)(1-x^4)(1-x^2)(1-x^2)} = \frac{x^3}{(1-x^2)(1-x^3)(1-x^4)}.$$

There are yet additional formulae for T_n, established by researchers. We list these below:

a. $T_n = \dfrac{6n^2 + 18n - 1}{288} + (-1)^{n+1}\dfrac{2n+3}{32} + \dfrac{c}{72}$

where $c = 7, -17, 1$, or 25 as n is congruent modulo 12 to (0 or 9), to $(1, 4, 5, 8)$, to (2, 7, 10 or 11), or to (3 or 6).

b. Given any number x, let $[x]$ denote the greatest integer function, and $\{x\}$ denote the nearest integer function. We can use these numbers to express T_n. Here

$$T_n = \left\{\frac{n^2}{12}\right\} - \left[\frac{n}{4}\right]\left[\frac{n+2}{4}\right].$$

c. Also, T_n is given by

$$T_n = \begin{bmatrix} \left\{\dfrac{n^2}{48}\right\} & \text{if } n \text{ is even} \\ \left\{\dfrac{(n+3)^2}{48}\right\} & \text{if } n \text{ is odd.} \end{bmatrix}$$

d. If $n \geq 4$ is even and r is defined by

$n = 12k + r$ $(4 \leq r \leq 14)$, then

$$T_n = \frac{n^2 - r^2}{48} + T_r.$$

If n is odd and r is defined by

$n = 12k + r, 1 \leq r \leq 11$, then

$$T_n = \frac{n(n+6) - r(r+6)}{48} + T_r.$$

If n is even, then, $T_{n+12} = T_n + \frac{n}{2} + 3$ and if n is odd then

$$T_{n+12} = T_n + \frac{n+9}{2}.$$

Let n be a positive integer and $p_3(n), p_2(n)$ denote the number of partitions of n into 3 and 2 parts respectively.

Then $T(n) = p_3(n) \sum_{1 \leq j \leq [\frac{n}{2}]} p_{2(j)}$.

The proofs of these statements are not given here. The reader can verify these statements for small values of n. For proofs, one may refer to the papers/articles on this topic given at the end of the book.

Lecture 13

Correction of Incorrectly Transmitted Messages

Abstract

In this lecture, we will develop the mathematical theory of sending correct messages through the Internet, using a code language common to computer systems. The problem of automatic detection and correction of errors in the messages, if any, is solved using graduate level mathematics.

13.1 Introduction

This is the age of computer networks. Information and messages are transmitted from one centre to another via satellites. Railway reservations, fax, e-mails are various instances of this exchange of information. The message to be sent is first transformed into the code language of the computer made up of computer alphabets – 0 and 1 only. It is also received in this code language and then transformed into the usual language.

Since the transmission process involves a complex system via satellites, errors are likely to occur in the received coded message. For example, the alphabet 0 in the transmitted message may be received as alphabet 1 due to some unknown defect in the system over which we may not have any control. Such a defect is called *noise*, which enters the transmission system. See Fig. 13.1. The received coded message must be automatically corrected by the computer itself at the receiving end, before it is transformed into the final received message. The purpose of this lecture is to explain the mathematics of error detection and correction in the coded language of the computer. Programmed instructions to the computer based on this mathematical theory will automatically allow the computer to detect errors and ultimately send a correct message.

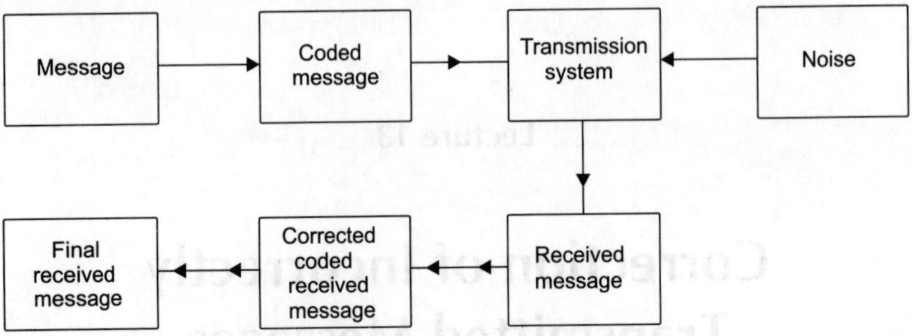

Fig. 13.1 Message transmission system

13.2 Coded Language

The computer knows only two alphabets 0 and 1. All the 26 English alphabets and their capital-letter forms, the integers 0 to 9, and other symbols used in common language such as ! , . , ( ), etc are coded in terms of standard codes of the computer. Each such code is a sequence of alphabets 0 and 1 called a *word*. The most commonly used standard code is the "American standard code of information interchange (ASCII)", which is a seven-bit code for each English alphabet, or numbers 0 to 9 etc. For example, $a \equiv 0\ 0\ 11\ 110$, $8 \equiv 1\ 0\ 0\ 00\ 11$ etc. in this code. Using this code, any English word or number, for example, can be transformed into the coded language of the computer. In general other n-bit codes, where n is a positive integer, can be constructed using only two alphabets 0 and 1. Thus the problem of transmitting English words or numbers etc. ultimately reduces to transmitting such n-bit codes from the set C_n of all such code words.

13.3 Error Detection

What precaution must be taken to ensure that the set C_n of all code words so constructed is convenient for detecting as well as for correcting the errors of transmission? First, an error of one alphabet in any member of C_n (zero changed to one or vice versa) should not produce another member of C_n. For example $8 = 1\ 0\ 0\ \underline{0}\ 011$ and $9 = 1\ 0\ 0\ \underline{1}\ 0\ 1\ 1$ in ASCII differ only at the fourth place. Hence if the transmitted word $1\ 0\ 0\ \underline{0}\ 0\ 11$ is received as $1\ 0\ 0\ \underline{1}\ 0\ 11$, then the error will not be suspected or detected and instead of the sent message "eight", a wrong message "nine" will be received. Thus ASCII code is not suitable for error detection of one alphabet. In our common language, if, the sent message "deed" is received as "dead", then since both are legitimate words of the English language, no error will be suspected at the receiving end. Hence we have

CONDITION 1: Any two code words of C_n must differ by at least two bit-places if an error in one bit-position is to be detected.

This criteria can be re-formulated by introducing the concept of a.

13.4 Distance Between Two Code Words

This is defined as the number of differing bit-positions between two code words of C_n.

For example, the code words for "a" and "8" in ASCII are 0011110 and 1000011 respectively and the distance between them,

$$d(0'01'1'1'10', 1'00'0'0'11') = 5$$

We have put "$'$" marks over differing bit-positions and counted the number of such marks. A better way is to write the two words one below another as follows. Then write 1 below the differing bit-positions and 0 below the identical bit-positions as shown below.

$$\begin{array}{ccccccc} 0 & 0 & 1 & 1 & 1 & 1 & 0 \\ 1 & 0 & 0 & 0 & 0 & 1 & 1 \\ \hline 1 & 0 & 1 & 1 & 1 & 0 & 1 \end{array}$$

Now count the number of 1s in the seven-bit word so obtained; call it the weight ϖ of the new word so formed. Then ϖ is the distance between the two words. In symbols,

$$d(0\,0\,11\,11\,0,\ 1\,0\,0\,0\,0\,11) = \varpi(0\,0\,11\,11\,0 * 1\,0\,0\,0\,0\,11)$$
$$= \varpi(1\,0\,1\,1\,1\,0\,1) = 5.$$

It may be verified that this definition of the distance between two words of same length (i.e., same number of bits) called Hamming distance is consistent with the general concept of distance which will be introduced in Lecture 14.

Our Condition 1 above can then be re-formulated as follows:

The minimum distance between any two code words of C_n must be ≥ 2 if a one-bit error has to be detected.

Generalising this result, we have the following provable

THEOREM 1: A code with a minimum distance of m+1 can detect at most m errors.

13.5 Error Correction

Having detected an error, we now turn to the problem of its correction. After receiving an erroneous word due to noise in the system, the system tries to locate that correct word in C_n which is " nearest " to the received incorrect word. This attempt may fail unless the minimum distance between any two code words of C_n is ≥ 3. Take an example. Suppose $\{11'0'0, 10'1'0\}$ are both standard code words in C_4. As they differ at two bit-places (second and third), the distance between them is 2 as required by Condition 1 above. Now if the received word after transmission is 1000, which is not a member of C_4, then the error is detected, but it cannot be corrected by the criteria of nearest code word in C_4; as both 1100 and 1010 are equidistant (at a distance 1) from 1000. So both 1100 and 1010 are possible correct words, and there is a confusion. Hence it is necessary that

CONDITION 2: If an error of one alphabet is to be corrected by the minimum distance criteria, then the distance between any two standard code words of C_n must be ≥ 3.

In general, we have the following provable

THEOREM 2: A code of minimum distance 2m+1 can correct m or fewer errors when the minimum distance criteria is applied.

13.6 Use of Group Theory

The theory of groups in algebra is found very useful in the problem of error correction posed above. In Section 13.3, for finding the distance between two code words of C_n, we introduced a binary algebraic operation " $*$ " on two code words of C_n. By writing 1 in the places of the differing corresponding bit-positions in the two words, and 0 in the places of identical corresponding bit-positions, we generate a new n-bit word. This word may or may not belong to C_n. We shall have to put this as an additional condition while formulating our set C_n of code words, if we want that the new word so f rmed from the two code words of C_n must also be a code word in C_n.

CONDITION 3: If $x, y \in C_n$, then $x * y$ must also belong to C_n.

If Condition 3 holds, then the binary operation $*$ on C_n is said to be closed in C_n.

Thus if Condition 3 holds, then the following properties hold for $*$ on C_n.

a. $x \in C_n, y \in C_n \Rightarrow x * y \in C_n$ ($*$ is closed).

b. $x * y = y * x$ for any $x, y \in C_n$ ($*$ is commutative).

c. $x * (y * z) = (x * y) * z$ for any x, y, z in C_n ($*$ is associative).

d. $x * x = (0, 0, 0, ...0) =$ "0", hence by Condition 3, $0 \in C_n$.

e. $x * 0 = x$ for any $x \in C_n$ (0 is the identity element for $*$).

Since 0 is an identity element, by property (e) it follows that each element x of C_n has a unique inverse and the inverse is x itself.

Thus by properties (a) to (e), C_n is a commutative group.

If we replace C_n above by S_n, the set of all n-bit words formed from the bits 0 and 1, and introduce the above binary operation $*$ on S_n, then we find that Condition 3 with C_n replaced by S_n holds automatically; it need not be assumed. The other properties (b) to (e) also hold. Thus (S_n, $*$) is also a commutative group. Since $C_n \subset S_n$ and (C_n, $*$) is also a group, C_n is called a subgroup of S_n.

13.7 Methods of Error Correction

Suppose the sent message $x \in C_n$ is transmitted as a message y which is in S_n but not in C_n.

Then one method of correction of the transmitted incorrect word y is to find its distance $d(y, z)$ for all elements z in C_n. Then that element $x \in C_n$ for which this distance $d(y, x)$ is least is the corrected word for the incorrect word y. Thus we find the code word x in C_n "nearest" to the incorrect word $y \notin C_n$; and take x as the correct word.

Another equivalent method of correction is to construct the coset $(y * C_n)$ whose members, all in S_n, are obtained by finding $y * z$ for each z in C_n. In short

$$(y * C_n) = \{(y * z) \in S_n / z \in C_n\}.$$

PROPOSITION: Let e be that member of the coset $(y * C_n)$ for which the weight (i.e., the number of 1s in e) is least (e is called the coset leader). Then $y * e$ is the correct word in C_n for the incorrect word $y \in S_n$.

PROOF: Let $e = y * x, x \in C_n$, so that $e \in (y * C_n)$ and $\varpi(e) < \varpi(z)$ for all $z \in (y * C_n) - \{e\}$, so that e is the element in $(y * C_n)$ of minimum weight. Now, using properties (a) to (e) of $*$

$$y * x = e \Rightarrow y * (y * x) = y * e$$

$$\Rightarrow (y * y) * x = y * e$$

$$\Rightarrow (0) * x = y * e$$

$$\Rightarrow x = y * e.$$

Thus x is determined from y by first finding the coset leader e.

According to a theorem in group theory, for any $a, b \in S_n$, the cosets (a $* C_n$) and (b $* C_n$), are either identical or mutually disjoint. Thus the possibility of locating x in any other coset different from $(y * C_n)$ is ruled out. Hence x is unique; which means x is the only correct word for the incorrect word y.

13.7.1 Procedure

The computer may be instructed to work out the following steps for a given subgroup of code words C_n in S_n.

1. List all members of S_n that are not in C_n.
2. For each z in the list of Step 1, find the coset $(z * C_n)$.
3. Locate that member e_z in each $(z * C_n)$ from Step 2 for which the weight is least.
4. Call e_z the coset leader of $(z * C_n)$.
5. Identify the received message y.
6. If $y \in C_n$, then y is the correct message.
7. If $y \notin C_n$, locate the coset leader C_y of that coset in Step 2 which contains y.
8. Find $x = y * C_y$.
9. x is the correct message for the incorrect message y.

Conclusion

Thus the problem of detecting and correcting the incorrectly transmitted message can be solved using elementary mathematics taught at the graduate level. The problem of constructing a group code C_n satisfying Conditions 1, 2, 3 has also been solved. (See the references). This lecture illustrates how important problems in computer science related to the Internet system, can be solved using group theory and allied concepts from mathematics.

Lecture 14

On Distance

Abstract

The reader might have already learnt about " distance" in the primary stage of education. On several occasions we use the term " distance" in our daily life. The term is used to describe quantitatively how far or near two cities, two planets, two trees, say, are from each other. It is also used abstractly in literature in terms like, distance between two ideas, distance between views of two persons etc. In this lecture we will try to understand the term " distance" in a mathematical sense.

14.1 Introduction

The name of the great mathematician Euclid and the subject of his study, geometry, go hand-in-hand with the history and development of mathematics. This celebrated mathematician, a citizen of Alexandria in Greece, lived during 330–270 BCE. He was the first mathematics professor in the Alexandria Museum. His lifetime overlapped that of the great philosopher Plato and it is likely that he received his training in Plato's Academy. Although Euclid and the development of geometry are so interlinked, he was not the first to discover geometry. There exists a vast history and body of knowledge of geometry before Euclid.

Euclid's name is synonymous to geometry because he is credited to have written a book which single-handedly helped in the systematic development of geometry. Euclid's monumental work, the *Elements* was a single chain of 467 propositions that, in part, encompasses plane and solid geometry. In the *Elements*, Euclid used a minimal set of assumptions called "postulates" and developed geometry. Hence *Elements* remained, for 2000 years, the most widely known example of a formal axiomatic system. It is because of this approach that Euclid is also known as a philosopher. For 2000 years, *Elements* was used as a textbook in several countries all over the world setting a record in textbook writing. Among various other aspects considered by Euclid in *Elements,* he provides a detailed discussion on the concept of distance. In this text, we will try to provide insights into some definitions of the distance c ncept and how it led to the development of different geometries.

14.2 What is Distance?

First let us consider what it means when we talk about the distance between two points A and B on a straight line. It is easy to understand that there are infinite number of ways for one to go from A and reach B. An infinite number of continuous graphs can be drawn between points A and B. Of all these paths, it is known that the shortest path is the straight line joining the points A and B. The length of this shortest curve between A and B is known as the distance between A and B. Observe that the distance between A and B is a unique number. In mathematical terms, if x and y are the distances of A and B respectively from the origin O as given in Fig. 14.1, then the distance between A and B is given by $|y - x|$ or $|x - y|$.

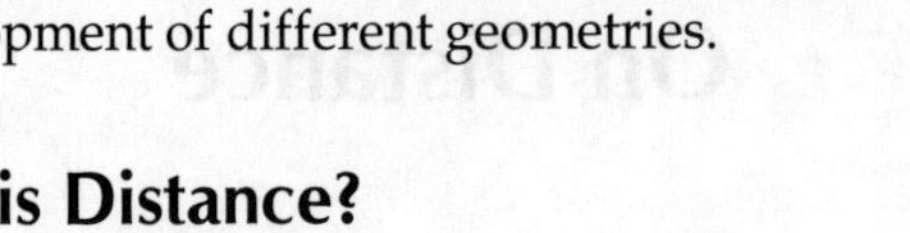

If OA $= x$, OB $= y$ then AB $=$ BA $= |y - x| = |x - y|$.

Fig. 14.1

Let us bring out the nature of the term "distance between two given points" as defined by Euclid. If A, B and C are any three points in a plane, then we have the following observations:

i. the "distance" is always a non-negative real number;

ii. the distance between the points A and B is zero if and only if A coincides with B;

iii. the distance from A to B is the same as the distance from B to A;

iv. the sum of the distances between A and B and B and C is greater than or equal to the distance between points A and C.

These four observations determine the nature of the term "distance" in Euclidean geometry. We can now present these observations in terms of a proper mathematical setting, i.e., in an axiomatic setting.

14.3 Axioms of "Distance"

Let x, y, z be any three elements of a non-empty set X. Let d: $X \times X \to R$ be a mapping satisfying the following axioms,

i. $d(x, y) \geq 0$ for all $x, y \in X$;

ii. $d(x, y) = 0$ if and only if $x = y$;

iii. $d(x, y) = d(y, x)$ (symmetry principle);

iv. $d(x, y) + d(y, z) \geq d(x, z)$, for all $x, y, z \in X$ (triangle inequality).

Whenever the mapping d satisfies the axioms (i) to (iv), we say that d is a metric on X (i.e., d stands for distance).

Thus, we have obtained here an abstract setting of the concept of distance. Naturally, Euclid's "distance" is a particular case of the generalised form of the "distance" concept. This statement also suggests that given two points on a line, Euclid "distance" is not the only distance—there can be many more "distances" between them. We will illustrate this fact from the following examples.

14.4 Examples on the Real Line *R*

1. Let x, y, z be real numbers on R. Consider the mapping $d(x, y) = |x - y|$ in Euclidean geometry. It is easy to observe that d satisfies all the four axioms stated above. We conclude that $d(x, y) = |x - y|$ is a "distance"—this is the distance we use in traditional geometry.

2. Let $d(x, y) = |x - y|$ be the distance given in (1) above. Define

$$d_1(x, y) = \frac{d(x, y)}{1 + d(x, y)}, x, y \in R$$

Let us verify if d_1 satisfies the axioms of a metric. Clearly

i. $d_1(x, y) \geq 0$;

ii. $d_1(x, y) = 0$ if and only if $x = y$, and

iii. $d_1(x, y) = d_1(y, x)$.

To verify the last axiom, we have

$$d_1(x, y) + d_1(y, z) = \frac{d(x, y)}{1 + d(x, y)} + \frac{d(y, z)}{1 + d(y, z)}$$

$$\geq \frac{d(x,y)+d(y,z)}{1+d(x,y)+d(y,z)}$$

$$= \frac{1}{1+\dfrac{1}{d(x,y)+d(y,z)}}$$

$$\geq \frac{1}{1+\dfrac{1}{d(x,z)}} = \frac{d(x,z)}{1+d(x,z)}$$

$$= d_1(x,z).$$

Thus d_1 is also a distance function and it measures the distance between any two points x, y on R. Further note that $d \neq d_1$. Observe that by using d_1, we can now define another metric, d_2 as follows.

$$d_2(x,y) = \frac{d_1(x,y)}{1+d_1(x,y)}, x, y \in R;$$

and repeat the proof given above for d_1. Hence, we prove that d_2 is also a function on $R \times R$. Notice that a sequence of distance functions, namely $(d_3, d_4, d_5, ..)$, can be formulated. This fact suggests that between any two points on a line R, we can have infinite number of distances; the traditional " distance " in Euclidean geometry is only one of these.

3. We can also verify that the following definitions of d provide us some additional examples of distance functions on the real line:

   i. $d(x,y) = \sqrt{|x-y|}$;

   ii. $d_1(x,y) =$ minimum of $\{1, d(x,y)\}$, where $d(x,y) = |x-y|$;

   iii. $d(x,y) = \left|\dfrac{x}{1+|x|} - \dfrac{y}{1+|y|}\right|$.

14.5 Hamming Distance

Consider a cuboid of unit dimension. It has eight corners (Fig. 14.2). Let A be the set of these eight points given by their coordinates.

Hence we have

$$A = \{(1,0,0),(0,1,0),(0,0,1),(1,0,1),(0,1,1),(1,1,1,),(0,0,0)\}.$$

Define for any $x, y \in A$,

$d(x,y) =$ number of places where x and y in A have different entries in their coordinates.

For example, $d((1,0,0),(0,1,0)) = 2$ since the coordinate entries in two places are different. Also, $d((1,0,0),(1,1,1)) = 2$.

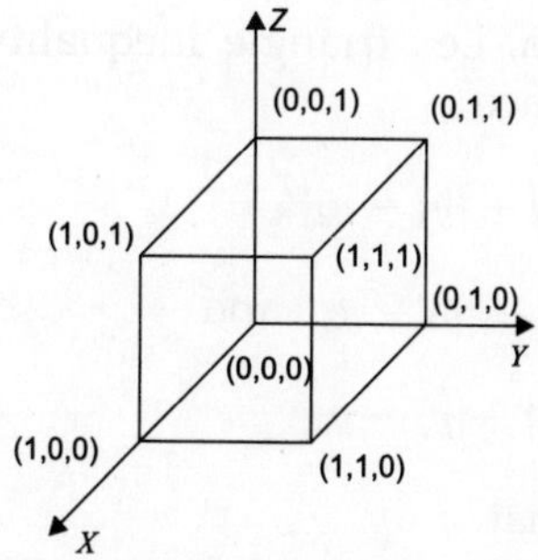

Fig. 14.2 A cuboid of unit dimension

It is observed that all the four axioms hold for this distance. We claim that d defines a "distance". This distance is known as the "Hamming distance" function. It has several applications in communication technology. One of these applications related to error detection and correction has already been discussed in Chapter 13.

14.6 Examples on $X = R^2$

Consider the triangle PQR (Fig. 14.3) in a plane. Let P $= (x_1, y_1)$, and Q $= (x_2, y_2)$.

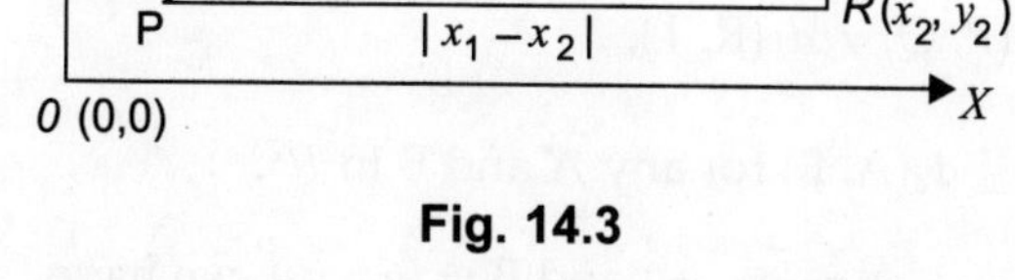

Fig. 14.3

Set

$$d_1(\text{P}, \text{Q}) = d_1((x_1, y_1), (x_2, y_2)) = \sqrt{|x_1 - x_2|^2 + |y_1 - y_2|^2}. \tag{1}$$

It is not difficult to show that d_1 satisfies the four axioms of distance. In fact, here geometrically d_1 (P, Q) is the length of the hypotenuse PQ.

Another distance function between the points P and Q is defined as

$$d_2\ (\text{P}, \text{Q}) = d_2((x_1, y_1), (x_2, y_2)) = |x_1 - x_2| + |y_1 - y_2|. \tag{2}$$

It is easy to verify axioms (i), (ii) and (iii) of distance.

For the fourth axiom, i.e., triangle inequality, let any point T have coordinates (x_3, y_3). Hence

$d_2(\mathrm{P}, \mathrm{Q}) = |x_1 - x_2| + |y_1 - y_2|$;

$d_2(\mathrm{P}, \mathrm{T}) = |x_1 - x_3| + |y_1 - y_3|$; and

$d_2(\mathrm{Q}, \mathrm{T}) = |x_2 - x_3| + |y_2 - y_3|$.

We can now prove that

d_2 (P, Q) $+d_2$ (Q, T) $\geq d_2$ (P, T), for all P, Q, T in R^2.

We now have two distance functions d_1 and d_2. We prove below a few properties of d_1 and d_2.

1. If d_2 (P, Q) $= d_2$ (R, T) then is it true that d_1 (P, Q) $= d_1$ (R, T)?

   The answer is that it is not true.

   For the proof, one counter-example is enough.

   Let P (5, 4), Q (1, 2), R (4, −3) and T (−2, −3) be the points in R^2.

   Here, d_2 (P, Q) $= d_2((5,4),(1,2)) = |5-1| + |4-2| = 6$,

   d_2 (R, T) $= d_2((4,-3),(-2,-3)) = |4+2| + |-3+3| = 6$.

   Hence $d_2(\mathrm{P}, \mathrm{Q}) = d_2(\mathrm{R}, \mathrm{T})$. Now

   $$d_1(\mathrm{P}, \mathrm{Q}) = d_1((5,4),(1,2)) = \sqrt{(5-1)^2 + (4-2)^2} = \sqrt{20},$$

   $$d_1(\mathrm{R}, \mathrm{T}) = d_1((4,-3),(-2,-3)) = \sqrt{(4+2)^2 + (-3+3)^2} = 6.$$

   Hence $d_1(\mathrm{P}, \mathrm{Q}) \neq d_1(\mathrm{R}, \mathrm{T})$.

2. d_1 (A, B) $\leq d_2$(A, B) for any A and B in R^2.

   When A $= (x_1, y_1)$ and B $= (x_2, y_2)$, we have

   $$d_1(\mathrm{A}, \mathrm{B}) = \sqrt{(x_1 - x_2)^2 + (y_1 - y_2)^2}, \text{ and}$$
   $$d_2(\mathrm{A}, \mathrm{B}) = |x_1 - x_2| + |y_1 - y_2|.$$

   We know from algebra, the inequality $\sqrt{a^2 + b^2} \leq |a| + |b|$ for any a, b in R. The result follows.

14.7 Taxicab Geometry

In this chapter, we will not discuss the Euclidean distance d_1 in great detail since it is assumed that the reader is aware of many properties of d_1 and its applications. Rather, we propose to present some examples which involve the distance d_2. In particular, some graphs have been presented so as to provide insight into the working of the distance d_2 in standard geometrical figures. One can see that the definition of the distance d_2 is like how a taxi travels in a city. Hence with d_2 we have what we all "*taxicab geometry*". Well-known author, Eugene F Krause in his book *Taxicab Geometry, An Adventure in Non-Euclidean Geometry* takes readers for a city ride and brings out beautifully the niceties of this journey [4]. Read also [1, 6].

It is known that a circle is a locus of a point which remains at a constant distance from a fixed point. Here the constant distance is called the radius of a circle, say r and the fixed point is called the centre of a circle, say (a, b). In mathematical symbols, we can write this statement in the form

$$\odot = \{P(x, y) : d((x, y), (a, b)) = r\}.$$

i. In case of d_1 – the distance given by (1), we have

$$\odot = \{P(x, y) : d_1((x, y), (a, b)) = r\}.$$

Let us consider a particular circle namely $(a, b) = (0, 0)$ and $r = 1$, i.e., a unit circle with centre at the origin.

Then $\odot = \{P(x, y) : d_1((x, y), (0, 0)) = \sqrt{x^2 + y^2} = 1\}$.

This circle is represented in Fig. 14 4.

This is a familiar picture of a circle.

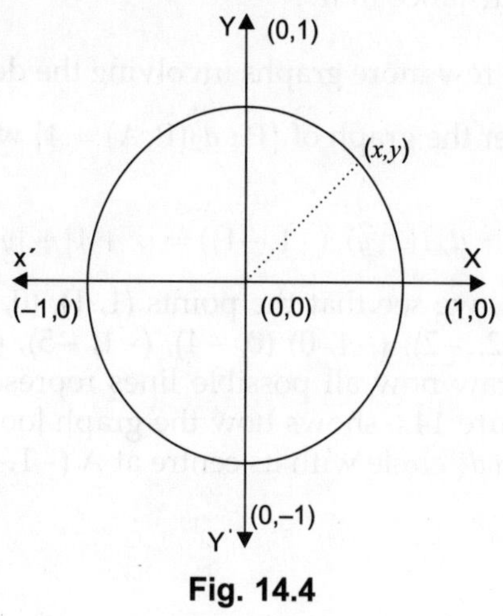

Fig. 14.4

ii. We now draw a geometrical figure of a circle when "distance" is d_2 as in (2). Clearly the unit circle is given by a set of points.

$$\odot = \{P(x, y) : d_2((x, y), (0, 0)) = 1\}.$$
$$= \{P(x, y) : |x| + |y| = 1\}.$$

It is easy to verify that the points (1, 0), (0, 1), (−1, 0), (0, −1) satisfy the equation $|x| + |y| = 1$ and hence are points on the circle. $|x| + |y| = 1$ represents four lines $x + y = 1$, $-x + y = 1$, $x - y = 1$ and $-x - y = 1$. When we draw these lines, we get the graph of this circle as in Fig. 14.5.

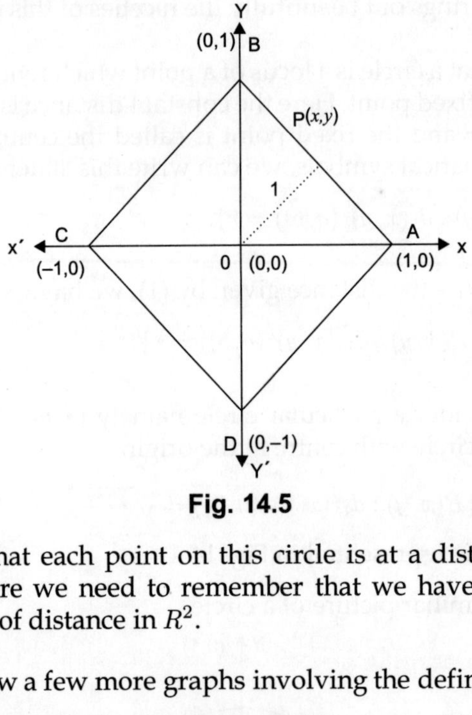

Fig. 14.5

Observe that each point on this circle is at a distance 1 from the origin. Here we need to remember that we have taken d_2 as the definition of distance in R^2.

iii. Let us draw a few more graphs involving the definition of d_2.

Let us consider the graph of $\{P : d_2(P, A) = 4\}$ with $A(-1, -1)$ in R^2. By definition,

$$d_2(P, A) = d_2((x, y), (-1, -1)) = |x + 1| + |y + 1| = 4.$$

By inspection, we see that the points (1, 1), (0, 2), (2, 0) (−1, 3) (3, −1), (−2, 2) (2, −2), (−4, 0) (0, −4), (−1, −5), (−5, −1) are on the graph. We draw now all possible lines represented by the above equation. Figure 14.6 shows how the graph looks. We can say that it represents a d_2 circle with its centre at A (−1,−1), and radius 4.

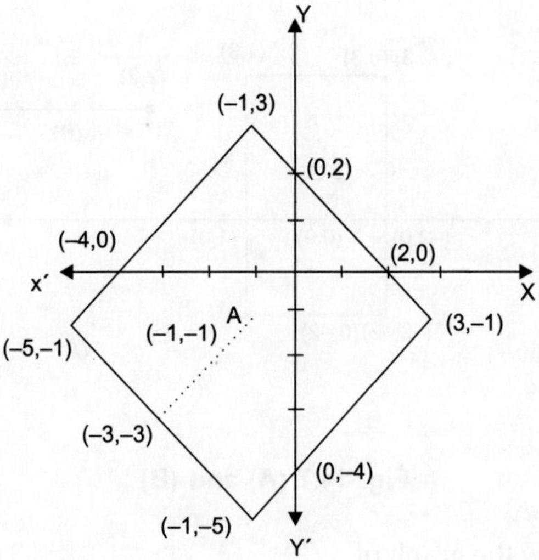

Fig. 14.6

iv. Draw the graph of

$$\{P(x, y) : d_2(P, A) + d_2\ (P, B) = d_2\ (A, B),$$

with $A(-2, 4)$ and $B(1, -3)\}$.

Clearly

$$\{P(x, y) : d_2(P, A) + d_2(P, B) = d_2(A, B)\}$$

$$= \{P(x, y) : d_2\ ((x, y), (-2, 4)) + d_2\ ((x, y), (1, -3))$$

$$= d_2\ ((-2, 4), (1, -3))\}$$

$$= \{P(x, y) : |x + 2| + |y - 4| + |x - 1| + |y + 3| = |-3| + |7| = 10\}.$$

The equation in the brackets need to be resolved by taking appropriate expressions of absolute values and then drawing these lines. Some points on the graph are $(-2, 3)$, $(-2, 0)$, $(-2, 2)$, $(1, -2)$, $(1, 0)$, $(1, 3)$. Figure 14.7(A) provides us the graph.

Let, in the above example, A(2, 2) and B(6, 2) be the given points. Then we have, as before, the graph

$$= \{P(x, y) : |x - 2| + |y - 2| + |x - 6| + |y + 2| = |2 - 6| + |2 - 2| = 4\}$$

The graph is a line joining (2, 2), (6, 2) given in Fig. 14.7(B).

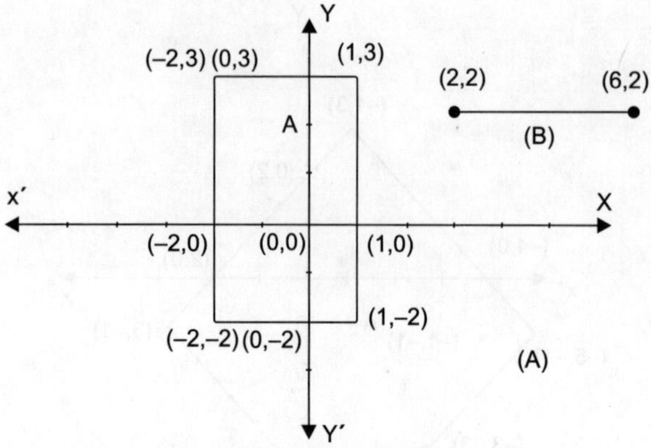

Fig. 14.7 (A) and (B)

v. Let us draw the graph of

$$\{P(x, y) : d_2\ (P, A) = d_2\ (P,B) \text{ with } A\ (0,0) \text{ and } B(2,4)\}.$$

Here the graph is the set of points

$$\{P(x, y) : d_2\ ((x, y), (0, 0)) = d_2\ ((x, y), (2, 4))\}$$

$$= \{P(x, y) : |x| + |y| = |x - 2| + |y - 4|\}.$$

Note that points (2, 1) and (0, 3) are on the graph. Further, all points $(x, 1), x \geq 2$ and $(x, 3), x \leq 0$ satisfy the equation and hence are on the graph. All points on the line $x + y = 3, 0 \leq x \leq 2$, are on the graph. The final graph is as given in Fig. 14.8.

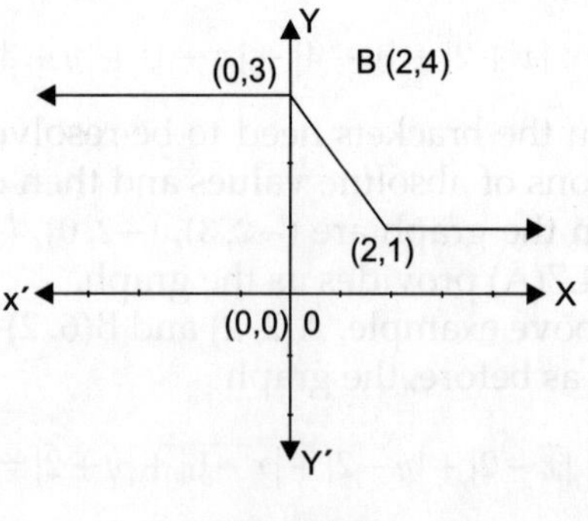

Fig. 14.8

vi. Draw the graph of

$$\{P(x, y) : d_2(P, A) = 2d_2\ (P,B) \text{ with } A(-3, 0) \text{ and } B(1,2)\}.$$

The graph is the set of points

$$\{P(x, y) : d_2((x, y), (-3, 0)) = 2d_2((x, y), (1, 2))\}$$
$$= \{P(x, y) : |x + 3| + |y| = 2[|x - 1| + |y - 2|]\}.$$

We leave it to the readers to draw the graph.

14.8 d_2-Ellipse

We know that the definitions of the well-known curves, namely, parabola, ellipse and hyperbola involve the concept of a " distance ". We are also familiar with their graphs when we use the " distance " definition given in (1). It is natural to expect that when d_1 in (1) is replaced by d_2 in (2), the new figures will become interesting. We provide below a few examples involving these graphs.

We know that a d_1-ellipse is a locus of a point whose sum of distances from two fixed points (called foci) is a constant.

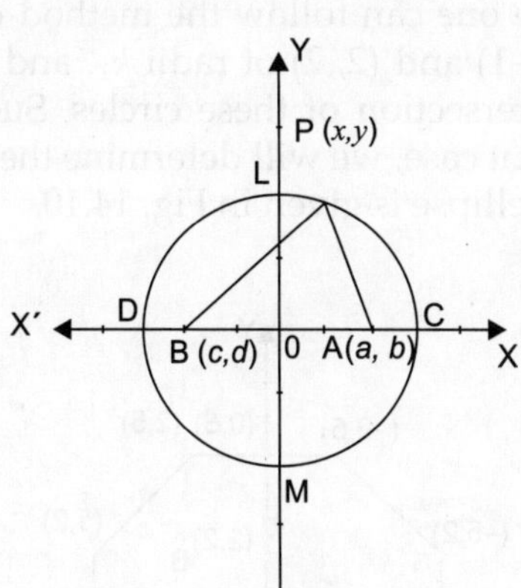

Fig. 14.9 d_1-ellipse: The points A and B are foci.

To get the d_1-ellipse we find the path followed by P such that PA + PB = constant, i.e.

$$\sqrt{(x - a)^2 + (y - b)^2} + \sqrt{(x - c)^2 + (y - d)^2} = \text{constant.}$$

Given A(a, b) and B(c, d), we will describe a method of drawing an ellipse. Suppose that the constant on the right side is k. Partition k into two positive numbers, say $k_1 + k_2 = k$. Draw a circle of radius k_1 with centre (a, b) and another one of radius k_2 with centre (c, d). The circles will generally intersect at two points. These points of intersection are the points on the ellipse. For, if P is the point of intersection, PA= k_1

and PB= k_2 making PA + PB = $k_1 + k_2 = k$. Keep on partitioning k into two parts and draw circles as mentioned earlier. Once we have enough number of points we can join these by a smooth curve.

There are other methods of drawing d_1-ellipses given in books on introductory coordinate geometry.

We now define d_2-ellipse as a locus of a point P(x, y) such that d_2(P, A) + d_2(P, B) = constant where A and B are given fixed points i.e., foci. Hence

$$d_2\text{-ellipse} = \{P(x,y) : d_2(P,A) + d_2(P,B) = \text{constant}\}.$$

Draw the d_2-ellipse, for A(−2, −1) and B(2, 2) and k = 13. Thus

$$d_2\text{-ellipse} = \{P(x,y) : d_2((x,y),(-2,-1)) + d_2((x,y),(2,2) = 13\}$$

$$= \{P(x,y) : |x+2| + |y+1| + |x-2| + |y-2| = 13\}.$$

By inspection (0, 5), (0, −4), (5, 0), (−5, 0), (5, 2), (2, 5), (−2, 5) (−5, 2), (−2, −4), (2, −4) are points on the graph. In fact, many more points can be obtained by inspection itself.

To obtain an ellipse one can follow the method of drawing d_2-circles around the foci (−2, −1) and (2, 2) of radii k_1, and k_2, whose sum is 13 and determine the intersection of these circles. Such points are on the d_2-ellipse. In the present case, we will determine the points by inspection only. The graph of d_2-ellipse is given in Fig. 14.10.

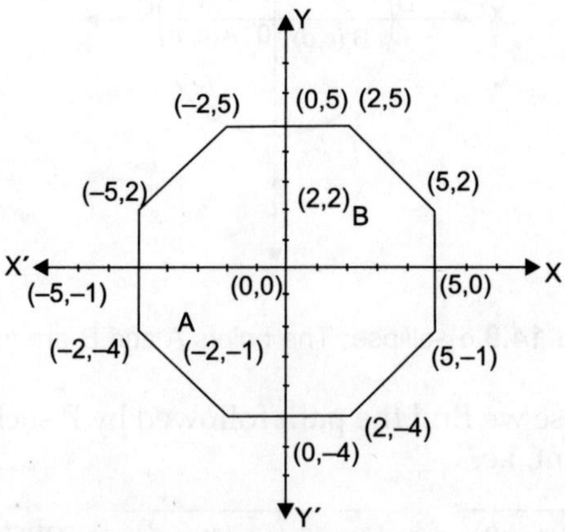

Fig. 14.10 d_2-Ellipse

14.9 d_2-Hyperbola

As opposed to an ellipse, in a hyperbola we have PA−PB = constant, (Refer to Fig. 14.11) where points A and B are given and P is a variable point. The locus is a d_1-hyperbola. If we take the same constant and consider PB−PA = constant, then, we obtain the other branch of the hyperbola. Hence for a complete description of a hyperbola, we need |PA−PB| = constant. The d_1-hyperbola has a graph as shown in Fig. 14.11.

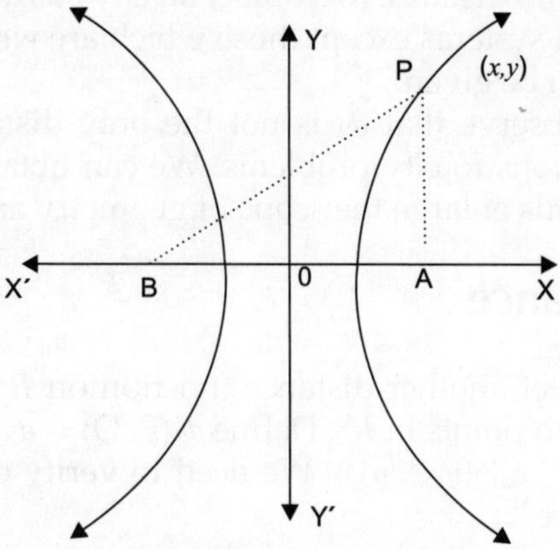

Fig.14.11 d_1-hyperbola

Now, let us consider a d_2-hyperbola

$$\{\text{P}(x, y) : |d_2(\text{P, A}) - d_2(\text{P, B})| = 3\}$$

where A(−3, −1) and B(2, 2) are fixed points. The graph of this hyperbola is given in Fig. 14.12.

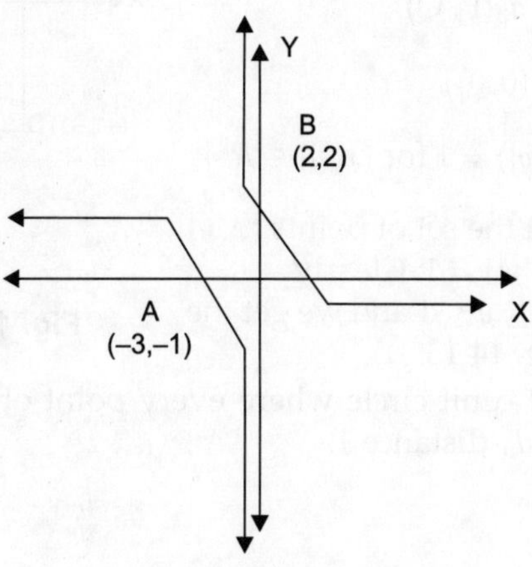

Fig. 14.12 d_2-hyperbola

Readers are advised to verify, by drawing two d_2-circles of radii k_1 and k_2 and centres at A and B, if the theory described in case of the ellipse in the previous section, works here. In this case we need to obtain $k_1 - k_2 = 3$ or $k_2 - k_1 = 3$ and determine their points of intersection.

It has been found that taxicab geometry is a useful model for urban geography. In urban areas, people and taxies travel along streets and lanes. When we say that the post office in a city is closer than the bus stand from a house, we take into account d_2-distance and not the distance as a crow flies, i.e., d_1-distance (of course, no city has an ideal rectangular framework of road systems except those which are well-planned). Many other examples can be given.

One can also observe that d_2 is not the only distance function that possesses applications to city problems. We can obtain new definitions of distances and thus enlarge the scope of geometry and applications.

14.10 d_3-distance

We define below yet another distance function on R^2. Let P(x_1, y_1) and Q(x_2, y_2) be any two points in R^2. Define d_3(P, Q) $= d_3((x_1, y_1), (x_2, y_2)) =$ maximum of $(|x_1 - x_2|, |y_1 - y_2|)$. We need to verify that d_3 satisfies the axioms of " distance".

With d_3-distance, let us draw a circle whose centre is at Q(a, b) and radius is r. Then the circle is a set

$$\odot = \{P(x, y) \in R^2 : d_3((x, y), (a, b)) = r\}$$

$$= [(x, y) \in R^2 : \max\{|x - a|, |y - b|\} = r].$$

As a particular case, let $(a,b) = (0, 0)$ and $r = 1$. Then we have a unit circle given by

$$\odot = \{P(x, y) : d_3(\text{P}, \text{Q})$$

$$= d_3\left((x, y), (0, 0)\right)$$

$$= \max(|x|, |y|) = 1 \text{ for } (x, y) \in R^2\}.$$

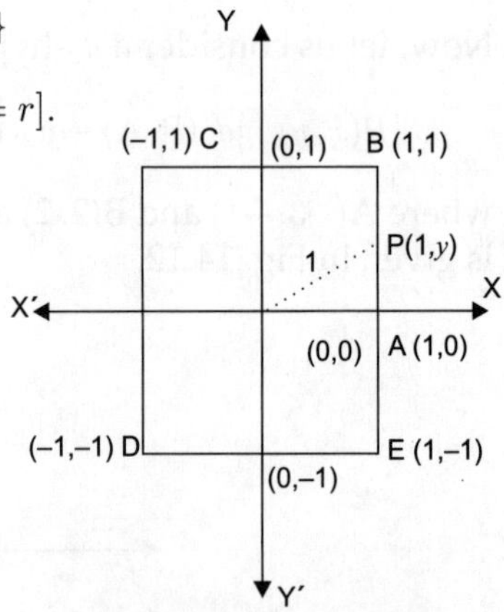

Fig. 14.13 d_3-distance

Hence we collect the set of points (x, y) such that max $(|x|, |y|) = 1$. Clearly $-1 \leq x \leq 1$ and $-1 \leq y \leq 1$ and we get the graph shown in Fig. 14.13.

Thus we get a d_3-unit circle where every point of this circle is away from the origin by d_3-distance 1.

14.11 Distance in a Discrete Set

We now study a general set in which " distance " ideas can be introduced. Let $X = (x_1, x_2, x_3, ..., x_n, ...)$ be a sequence of numbers, real or complex.

$$\text{Define} \quad d(x_i, x_j) = \begin{cases} 1 + \dfrac{1}{i+j} & \text{when } i \neq j; \\ 0, & \text{when } i = j. \end{cases}$$

Clearly i. $d(x_i, x_j) \geq 0$, for $i, j \in N$;

ii. $d(x_i, x_j) = 0$, iff $i = j$;

iii. $d(x_i, x_j) = d(x_j, x_i)$, $i, j \in N$;

and

iv. $1 + \dfrac{1}{i+j} + 1 + \dfrac{1}{j+k} \geq 1 + \dfrac{1}{i+k}$, for all $i, j, k, \in N$.

Hence d indeed defines the " distance " function. Define a ball in X by,

$$B(x_0, r) = \{x; d(x, x_0) \leq r, x_0 \text{ is the centre, } r \text{ is the radius}\}.$$

$$B\left(x_i, \frac{1}{2}\right) = \left\{x_j \in X; d(x_j, x_i) \leq \frac{1}{2}\right\}$$

$$= \left\{x_j \in X; 1 + \frac{1}{i+j} \leq \frac{1}{2}\right\}.$$

Clearly, this is impossible when $i \neq j$. Further, for $j = i$

$$B\left(x_i, \frac{1}{2}\right) = \left\{x_j \in X; 0 \leq \frac{1}{2}\right\}.$$

Hence we find that the ball contains a single point x_i, the centre of the ball.

Consider another ball having its centre at x_n and radius $1 + \dfrac{1}{2n}$. We have now

$$B\left(x_n, 1 + \frac{1}{2n}\right) = \left\{x_j \in X; d(x_n, x_j) \leq 1 + \frac{1}{2n}\right\}$$

$$= \left\{x_j \in X; 1 + \frac{1}{n+j} \leq 1 + \frac{1}{2n}\right\}$$

the inequality in the bracket namely $\dfrac{1}{n+j} \le \dfrac{1}{2n}$ holds for $j = 1, 2, \ldots.., n$. Hence the given ball contains the element $x_j \in X$ i.e. $x_1, x_2, \ldots., x_{n-1}$ and x_n.

Many of such ideas enrich the branch of modern analysis, a branch of mathematics.

14.12 Generalised Circles

We now define a much more general distance function. For $1 \le p < \infty$, define the distance between the points P (x_1, y_1) and Q (x_2, y_2) by

$$D_p(\text{P}, \text{Q}) = [|x_1 - x_2|^p + |y_1 - y_2|^p]^{1/p} \qquad (p \text{ is a + ve integer})$$

Clearly D_1 (P, Q) $= |x_1 - x_2| + |y_1 - y_2|$ and

$$D_2\ (\text{P}, \text{Q}) = \sqrt{|x_1 - x_2|^2 + |y_1 - y_2|^2}.$$

Note that in our previous discussions, we have taken $D_1 = d_2$ and $D_2 = d_1$. In an interesting paper [2], Euler Russel and Sadek Javad have considered the values $p = 3, 4, 5, \ldots.$

Let $1 \le p < \infty$ and $r > 0$. The set $\{(x, y) \in R^2; |x|^p + |y|^p = r^p\}$ is called a generalised circle with centre at the origin and radius r. Denote this circle by $C_p(r)$.

If $p = \infty$, the distance between $\text{P}(x_1, y_1)$ and $\text{Q}(x_2, y_2)$ is given by

$$D_\infty\ (\text{P}, \text{Q}) = \max(|x_1 - x_2|, |y_1 - y_{2.}|).$$

From the notation $C_p(r)$, we find that $C_p(1)$ denotes the unit generalised circle. For $p = 1, 2, 3, \ldots$, we get unit generalised circles. These are shown in Fig. 14.14

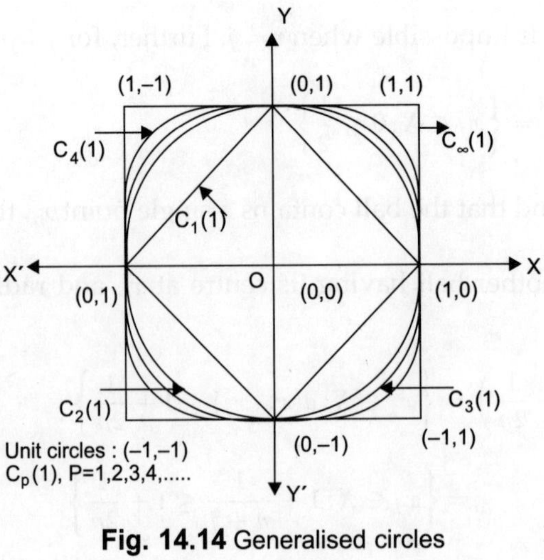

Fig. 14.14 Generalised circles

Observe that $C_2(1)$ denotes the traditional unit circle. Figure 14.14 illustrates that as $p \to \infty,\ C_1 \to C_\infty(1)$.

Conclusion

By the end of this chapter, we realise that we can think much beyond the traditional concept of the distance known to us. This fact leads to many interesting generalisations. Reference [4] provides us taxicab geometry, and its applications in urban society. Particularly, student readers can prepare projects based on this chapter The readers may also suggest new situations wherein the unknown distance definitions work.

Lecture 15

Modelling with Differential Equations

Abstract

The purpose of this chapter is to illustrate with examples that many important realistic problems from a variety of branches in science and engineering can be solved by skillfully formulating their mathematical models using simple easily solvable ordinary differential equations. Three problems from medical sciences have been solved this way for illustration.

15.1 Introduction

Many realistic problems from various walks of life, outside the world of mathematics, can be brought into it by

i. mathematical representations,

ii. solution using well-developed mathematical techniques, and then finally,

iii. the interpretation of the solutions in terms of the non-mathematical language of the problem.

This art is known as mathematical modelling and it makes mathematics useful in solving a variety of problems in several branches of knowledge, thus justifying the claim that mathematics is the mother science feeding all other subjects.

To illustrate this point, a variety of real-world problems solvable by using simple ordinary differential equations have been discussed in the following two books:

i. Burghs, D N and M S Barrie *Modelling with Differential Equations.*

ii. Braun M, C S Coleman and D A Drew. *Differential Equation Models.*

We shall discuss some.

15.2 Problems modelled by *dy/dt* = *ky*

In these problems k is a constant. This is a statement that says that the rate of increase of a variable quantity y over time is proportional to y itself. This simple model works for a variety of problems and the results obtained, based on the solution

$$y(t) = y(t_0) \exp k(t - t_0), \tag{1}$$

are found to be in good agreement with reality. Here $y(t_0) = y_0$ is the value of y at $t = t_0$. If y decreases as t increases, then the equation becomes $dy/dt = -ky, k > 0$.

15.2.1 Population growth

Malthus postulated that the rate of increase of human population y is directly proportional to the population y itself. The population at time t is then known from (1) if the initial population at $t = 0$ is known. This model was used to estimate the population of USA for every ten years (and did so quite correctly) from 1790 to 1850 CE. Thus it worked well for 60 years.

15.2.2 Oil production

The rate of increase of world oil production y in million metric tons per year was assumed to be proportional to y itself. This equation was generally in agreement with the observed data during 1960–1966; when 1960 CE was taken as $t = 0$ with $y_0 = 1091$. Then the subsequent values of y for 1962, '64 and '66 were in good agreement with the observed values (approximately). So the oil production during 1968, '70 and '72 was predicted using equation (1) and the subsequent actual results were in good agreement with the results.

Similarly, the solution of the equation gave approximately good results during 1945 to 1970, against observed data.

15.2.3 Weight-loss

Over-weight people on diet and treatment gradually reduce their weight y. The time rate of decrease of weight y is assumed to be proportional to the weight y itself. What most people, both amateurs and professionals, are interested in is how long it will take to reduce the weight to a desired value advised by the doctor. This problem is solvable by equation (1).

15.3 Some Problems from Medical Sciences

We shall briefly mention three interesting problems.

- Determination of the time of death (especially in murder cases) from a post-mortem examination of the dead body, using Newton's law of cooling.
- Quantity and period of a periodic dose for a person requiring prolonged treatment with a desirable concentration of drug in the blood.
- Hemodialysis via an artificial kidney machines (dialyser).

15.3.1 Time of death

According to Newton's law of cooling, the rate of decrease of y, the excess temperature of the dead body over the surrounding known constant temperature y_s, is directly proportional to y itself. Initially at $t = 0$, (the commencement *of this* " zero " time is unknown), as soon as the murder takes place, the temperature of the body is the normal temperature of a living body, and thus y_0 is known. Subsequently the temperatures y_1, y_2 of the body are recorded at known clock hours, (say 11.30 PM and 12.30 AM), which are the temperatures at unknown times t_1 and t_2, although

$$t_2 - t_1 = T \tag{2}$$

is known. Noting that $dy/dt = -ky, k > 0$, and applying equation (1),

$$y(t_1) = y_1 = y_0 \exp(-kt_1), \tag{3}$$

$$y(t_2) = y_2 = y_0 \exp(-kt_2). \tag{4}$$

There are only three unknowns t_1, t_2, k in the three equations (2), (3), (4). If t_1 can be found, the time when the murder was committed can be estimated [say (11.30 PM $-t_1$) o'clock]. And t_1 can be obtained from (2), (3), (4) by simple algebra.

This method was successfully applied by Womack in 1887 to determine the time of death (he worked on 118 dead bodies of executed prisoners, whose time of death was therefore already known). He found the time to an accuracy within an error of maximum 25 minutes in the case of 57 prisoners out of 118. (See reference [3] at the end).

15.3.2 Drug absorption

A patient with prolonged illnesses like T.B, requires prolonged treatment of an effective drug, for example, penicillin in the case of T.B. A certain prescribed minimum concentration of this drug must be maintained in the blood for an effective cure. In actual practice, when a given dose is administered, the initial known concentration y_0 of the drug in the blood is high but then it decays gradually and becomes zero unless a second dose of the drug is administered on time. The proper adjustment of the dose and the period of the dose of a drug is therefore, a very important problem. It is again governed by equation (1) with K, *a* negative constant because the rate of decrease of the concentration y of a drug is proportional to y itself. If the concentration due to the initial dose is y_0, and the period between consecutive doses is T, then the concentration of y at time T after the first dose is

$$y(T_-) = y_0 e^{-K(T)}. \tag{5}$$

If the concentration is again increased by y_0 at $t = T_+$ by administering a second dose of the drug at $t = T_+$, the initial concentration at $t = T_+$ is,

$$y = y_0 + y_0 e^{-KT} \qquad \text{at } t = T_+ \tag{6}$$

This replaces y_0 in (5) and the concentration after time $2T_-$ is

$$y = y_0(1 + e^{-KT})e^{-K(T)} \tag{7}$$

After the administration of the third dose, the initial concentration at $2T_+$ is

$$y = y_0(1 + e^{-KT})e^{-KT} + y_0 \text{ at } t = 2T_+, \qquad \text{or}$$

$$y = y_0(1 + e^{-KT} + e^{-2KT}). \tag{8}$$

Continuing this way, the concentration after the $(n-1)$th dose at time nT_+ is

$$y(nT_+) = y_0(1 + e^{-KT} + e^{-2KT} + \ldots + e^{-nKT}). \tag{9}$$

Adding the terms of the geometrical progression on the right side of (9), we have

$$y(nT_+) = \frac{y_0(1 - e^{-(n+1)KT})}{1 - e^{-KT}} \tag{10}$$

For a prolonged treatment, n in (10) is very large. As, $n \to \infty$

$$y = y_0(1 + e^{-KT}). \tag{11}$$

Equation (11) gives the calculated concentration after many many doses in a prolonged treatment. The right side of (11) must match the desired minimum concentration y_d of the drug in the blood. So,

$$y_d = y_0(1 + e^{-KT}). \tag{12}$$

Equation (12) determines T for a given y_0 or gives y_0 for a given T.

15.3.3 Artificial Kidney Machine (Dialyser)

The main function of the kidney is to filter out waste material from the blood. In some instances, infection, diabetes, injury etc, the human kidney shuts down causing a build-up of toxic material in the blood. To purify this blood, an artificial kidney machine called a dialyser is used. The process of purification is called dialysis.

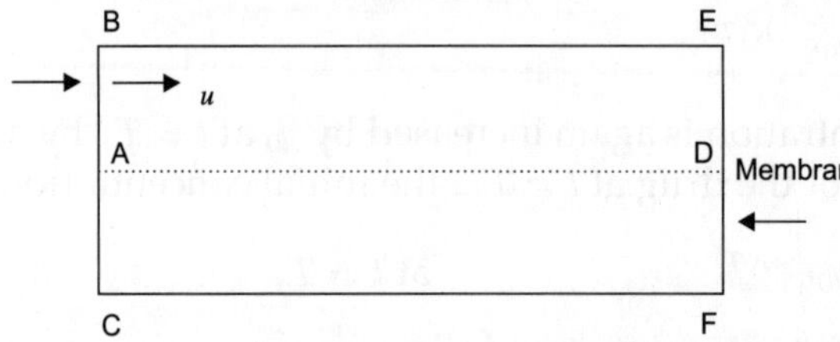

A dialyser has two compartments, separated by a perforated membrane, whose pores allow only the waste material from the blood to cross it but not the blood. When blood enters through AB and passes the upper compartment ADEB, the filtered waste material enters the lower compartment ACFD through the membrane $\overline{\text{AD}}$. The dialysate (chemicals used to draw toxins out of the blood and supply it with the necessary electrolytes) entering through $\overline{\text{DF}}$ in the lower compartment washes out this filtered waste through $\overline{\text{AC}}$. The filtration through $\overline{\text{AD}}$ occurs according to Fick's law.

> **Fick's Law:** The time rate of volume filtered per unit area of the membrane is proportional to the difference between the concentrations of waste material in the upper and lower compartment.

Taking the y axis along CAB with origin at C, the sides CAB and FDE are represented by $x = 0, x = L$. If $u(x)$ and $v(x)$ are respectively the concentrations of the waste in the upper and lower compartments and if Q_B is the volume flow rate across AB per unit breadth, then the mass conservation equation for ABED is that for a unit time and unit width, mass flow across AB = Mass flow through the membrane AD + Mass flow out through ED. Thus,

$$Q_B u(x) = K[u(x) - v(x)]dx \times 1 + Q_B u(x + dx), \tag{13}$$

where K is the proportionality constant in Fick's law. As $dx \to 0$, this leads to

$$Q_B \frac{du}{dx} = -K(u - v). \tag{14}$$

Similarly the mass conservation in ACDF gives,

$$-Q_D \frac{dv}{dx} = K(u - v) \tag{15}$$

where Q_D is the volume flow rate of the dialysate across $\overline{\text{FD}}$ per unit breadth. Equations (14) and (15) yield

$$\frac{dz}{dx} = -\alpha z \tag{16}$$

where $z = u - v, \alpha = K\left[\frac{1}{Q_B} - \frac{1}{Q_D}\right],$

which must be solved subject to the boundary conditions

$$u = u_0 \quad \text{at } x = 0, \qquad v = 0 = 0 \text{ at } x = L. \tag{17}$$

The method is to use the general solution of (16):

$$u - v = z = Ae^{-\alpha x}$$

in (14) and (15) and then solve for u and v using (17). The solution is

$$u = u_0 \left[\frac{e^{-\alpha L/Q_D} - e^{-\alpha x/Q_B}}{e^{-\alpha L/Q_D} - 1/Q_B}\right], \tag{18}$$

$$v = \frac{u_0}{Q_D}\left[\frac{e^{-\alpha L} - e^{-\alpha x}}{e^{-\alpha L/Q_D} - 1/Q_D}\right]. \tag{19}$$

The efficiency of the dialyser is determined by the clearance ratio

$$C_l = \frac{\text{Rate of waste mass removal}}{\text{Entering waste concentration}}$$

$$= \frac{1}{u_0} \int_0^L K(u(x) - v(x))dx$$

$$= \frac{Q_B}{u_0}(u_0 - u_L)$$

Thus

$$C_l = Q_B \left[\frac{1 - e^{-\alpha L}}{1 - (Q_B/Q_D)e^{-\alpha L}} \right]. \tag{20}$$

The experimental results, relating to urea, creatinine agree reasonably well with this result.

Equation (20) shows how the clearance ratio C_l depends upon the parameters Q_B (blood flux), Q_D (dialysate flux), K the Fick's constant and L the length of the dialyser. This information is important for the appropriate design and functioning of the dialyser.

Conclusion

The age of a buried fossil or that of the wooden throne of an emperor, important in a branch of history called anthropology, can be determined using Liby's invention of "carbon dating" (for which he got the Nobel prize). The mathematical formulation is again based on $dy/dt = Ky$.

Many such interesting realistic problems from various branches of knowledge can be solved using differential equations. Only a few simple samples are presented here. The two books mentioned during the introduction of this chapter give many more interesting examples based on a variety of ordinary differential equations. Some of these examples, based on systems of first or second order, linear or non-linear ordinary differential equations are discussed in Chapters 19, 20 and 21.

Models of many realistic problems, including industrial problems, are governed by partial differential equations (example: the well-known Laplace equation). But their discussion is beyond the scope of undergraduate students. It may be pursued during further reading.

Lecture 16

A Highway to Trigonometry I

Abstract

Trigonometry is generally taught at the higher secondary school level. The results in trigonometry are continuously used in almost all areas of mathematics. Most trigonometry heavily depends on the knowledge of Euclidean geometry. While these geometrical tools might help students understand many important results in this course, they may also prevent the realisation of possible generalisations and applications – in other words, it is not abstract enough to encompass the whole range of trigonometry.

The aim of the present lecture is to provide an alternative method (other than geometry) of achieving most of the results of trigonometry in a simple way. This alternative approach needs basic tools in calculus, basic course work in differential equations and a few results in mathematical analysis; and of course, we need to add a little patience. A prior knowledge of basic trigonometry makes the alternative approach more enjoyable. The alternative method is elegant, precise and rewarding. Needless to say that the creative faculty of our mind gets stimulated.

16.1 Introduction

We will consider the differential equations $x'' + x = 0$ and $x'' - x = 0$ with suitable initial conditions. These equations are linear, of second order, homogeneous and with constant coefficients. They possess solutions which exist on $(-\infty, \infty)$ and further, when initial conditions are given, they are unique. We know how to solve such equations explicitly and get solutions at hand for different applications. Here we do not aim to solve the equations explicitly. Rather we use analytical methods to study their qualitative properties. The methods are simple and elegant. Refer to [2].

16.2 Basic Relation in Trigonometry

Consider the differential equation

$$x'' + x = 0, \tag{1}$$

with initial conditions: $x(0) = 1, x'(0) = 0; x'(t) = \dfrac{dx}{dt}, t \in R$ and $'$ stands for differential.

For convenience, we can convert this equation into a system of equations by defining $x = x_1$ and $x' = x_1' = -x_2$. Thus, we have the system

$$x_1' = -x_2,\ x_2' = x_1. \tag{2}$$

and $x_1(0) = 1,\ x_2(0) = 0.$ (3)

The solution of the system (2) and (3) is a pair of functions $(x_1(t), x_2(t))$. These solutions exist uniquely on $(-\infty, \infty)$.

Multiply by x_1 the first equation of (2) and by x_2 the second equation of (2) on both sides and add to get

$$x_1 x_1' + x_2 x_2' = -x_2 x_1 + x_1 x_2 = 0.$$

Integration of both sides yields for $t \in (-\infty, \infty)$

$$x_1^2(t) + x_2^2(t) = c; \text{ (} c \text{ is a constant of integration).}$$

Now apply initial data at $t = 0$ to conclude that $c = 1$. Thus we get the first relation between x_1 and x_2, namely

$$x_1^2(t) + x_2^2(t) = 1; \quad t \in (-\infty, \infty). \tag{4}$$

The relation (4) suggests that

$$-1 \le x_1(t) \le 1 \text{ and } -1 \le x_2(t) \le 1, t \in (-\infty, \infty).$$

Further, when $x_1^2(t)$ is increasing, $x_2^2(t)$ is a decreasing function of t and vice-versa.

16.3 Addition Formulae

Let $\alpha \in R$ be arbitrary. We prove that the solution set $(x_1(t), x_2(t))$ of (2) and (3) possesses the properties, for any $\alpha \in R$:

$$x_1(t + \alpha) = x_1(t)x_1(\alpha) - x_2(\alpha)x_2(t), \text{ and} \tag{5}$$

$$x_2(t+\alpha) = x_1(t)x_2(\alpha) + x_1(\alpha)x_2(t), \quad t \in (-\infty, \infty). \tag{6}$$

To prove (5) and (6), we have two sets of solutions $(x_1(t), x_2(t))$ and $(x_1(t+\alpha), x_2(t+\alpha))$ of (2) with different initial data. These two sets of solutions are related by

$$x_1(t+\alpha) = c_1 x_1(t) + c_2 x_2(t), \tag{7}$$

and $$x_2(t+\alpha) = d_1 x_1(t) + d_2 x_2(t); \quad t \in (-\infty, \infty), \ \alpha \in R. \tag{8}$$

Here c_1, c_2, d_1 and d_2 are constants to be chosen appropriately. Clearly for $t = 0$, we have

$$x_1(\alpha) = c_1 x_1(0) + c_2 x_2(0) = c_1$$

and $x_2(\alpha) = d_1 x_1(0) + d_2 x_2(0) = d_1$.

We have used (3). Thus we have obtained the values of c_1 and d_1.

Further, differentiating (7) and (8), we have

$$\begin{aligned} x_1'(t+\alpha) &= c_1 x_1'(t) + c_2 x_2'(t) = -c_1 x_2(t) + c_2 x_1(t) \\ &= -x_2(t+\alpha), \end{aligned} \tag{9}$$

$$\begin{aligned} x_2'(t+\alpha) &= d_1 x_1'(t) + d_2 x_2'(t) = -d_1 x_2(t) + d_2 x_1(t) \\ &= x_1(t+\alpha). \end{aligned}$$

For $t = 0$, we get from (9), $-x_2(\alpha) = c_2$ and $x_1(\alpha) = d_2$.

Now substitute the values of c_1, d_1, c_2 and d_2 in (7) and (8). Observe that the resulting relations are (5) and (6). These relations are called "addition formulae". Following the above method, we can also prove that

$$x_1(t-\alpha) = x_1(t)x_1(\alpha) + x_2(t)x_2(\alpha); \tag{10}$$

$$x_2(t-\alpha) = -x_1(t)x_2(\alpha) + x_1(\alpha)x_2(t).$$

The relations (5), (6) and (10) are useful. For $\alpha = t$, we have

$$x_1(2t) = x_1^2(t) - x_2^2(t) = 2x_1^2(t) - 1 = 1 - 2x_2^2(t); \text{ and}$$

$$x_2(2t) = 2x_1(t)x_2(t).$$

For $\alpha = 2t$, we get

$$x_1(3t) = 4x_1^3(t) - 3x_1(t) \text{ and } x_2(3t) = 3x_2(t) - 4x_2^3(t).$$

For $t = 0$,

$$x_1(-\alpha) = x_1(\alpha) \text{ and } x_2(-\alpha) = -x_2(\alpha).$$

These relations prove that $x_1(t)$ is an even function and $x_2(t)$ is an odd function. Further, the relations (6) and (10) yield

$$x_1(t+\alpha)+x_1(t-\alpha)=2x_1(t)x_1(\alpha);$$

$$x_1(t+\alpha)-x_1(t-\alpha)=2x_2(t)x_2(\alpha); \text{ and}$$

$$x_2(t+\alpha)+x_2(t-\alpha)=2x_2(t)x_1(t);$$

$$x_2(t+\alpha)-x_2(t-\alpha)=2x_2(\alpha)x_1(t).$$

Many more familiar formulae can be derived by combining the above relations.

16.4 Periodic Solutions

We now show that there exists a positive number t_0 in R such that $x_1(t_0)=0$. Suppose that such a $t_0 \geq 0$ does not exist. We will then show that there is a contradiction. Since $x_1(0)=1$ and $x_1(t)$ is a continuous function, assume that $x_1(t)$ remains positive for $t \geq 0$. Hence in view of (2), $x_2'(t) \geq 0$ for $t \geq 0$. Thus $x_2(t)$ is an increasing function of t and $x_2(t) > 0$ for $t \geq 0$.

Let $T \geq 0$ be any arbitrary number. Consider the interval $0 \leq t \leq T$. Then we have

$$x_2(t)(T-t) \leq \int_t^T x_2(s)ds = \int_t^T -x_1'(s)ds = x_1(t)-x_1(T) \leq 2. \quad (11)$$

For the left-side inequality in (11), we have used the increasing character of $x_2(t)$ and for the right-hand side inequality we have used the fact that $-1 \leq x_1(t) \leq 1$. Since T is arbitrary, it can be selected sufficiently large so as to make $x_2(t)(T-t)$ greater than 2. Hence this inequality leads to a contradiction. The conclusion is that there exists $t_0 > 0$ such that $x_1(t_0)=0$.

The result proved above has important consequences. We now show that there exists a positive number p such that

$$x_1(t+p)=x_1(t), x_2(t+p)=x_2(t), t \in R. \quad (12)$$

If the relations (12) hold, it will mean that the solutions $(x_1(t), x_2(t))$ of (2) and (3) are periodic with period p. We will now change notation and write $t_0 = t^*$. To establish (12), suppose that $t^* > 0$ and $x_1(t^*)=0$. That such a t^* exists is clear from the discussion given above. Hence from (4), we have $x_2(t^*)=1$. Now,

$$x_1(2t^*)=x_1^2(t^*)-x_2^2(t^*)=0-1=-1, \text{ and}$$

$$x_2(2t^*)=2x_1(t^*)x_2(t^*)=0. \text{ Further}$$

$$x_1(4t^*) = x_1^2(2t^*) - x_2^2(2t^*) = 1; \text{ and}$$
$$x_2(4t^*) = 2x_1(2t^*)x_2(2t^*) = 0.$$

In view of the relations (5) and (6), we now have

$$x_1(t + 4t^*) = x_1(t)x_1(4t^*) - x_2(t)x_2(4t^*) = x_1(t), \text{ and}$$

$$x_2(t + 4t^*) = x_2(t)x_1(4t^*) + x_2(4t^*)x_1(t) = x_2(t).$$

Thus, relations (12) hold if we choose $p = 4t^*$ which is positive.

We have now discovered that $p = 4t^*$ is a period for the functions $x_1(t)$ and $x_2(t)$. Clearly any integer multiple of p namely kp (k is an integer) is also a period of $x_1(t)$ and $x_2(t)$.

Now the question to be answered is: is $p = 4t^*$ itself the smallest period of $x_1(t)$ and $x_2(t)$? We will answer this question below. Consider the set of positive integers P defined by

$$P = \{p : x_1(t + p) = x_1(t), x_2(t + p) = x_2(t)\}.$$

We show that $p^* = glp\{P\}$ is also a period and that $p^* > 0$. By the definition of greatest lower bound, there exists a sequence $\{p_1, p_2, p_3, \ldots\}$ in P which converges to p^*. Since $x_1(t)$ is a continuous function, $x_1(t+p_n)$ tends to $x_1(t + p^*)$ as $n \to \infty$. Since $p_n \in P$, $x_1(t + p_n) = x_1(t)$ for $n = 1, 2, 3, \ldots$. The limit of the sequence $\{x_1(t + p_n)\}$ is $x_1(t)$ and hence $x_1(t + p^*) = x_1(t)$. Thus p^* is also a period and a member of P. Clearly $p^* \geq 0$. Now, suppose that $p^* = 0$. Then

$$x_2(p_n) - x_2(0) = 0, n = 1, 2, 3, \ldots \text{ and,}$$

$$x_2'(0) = \lim_{n\to\infty} \frac{x_2(p_n) - x_2(0)}{p_n - 0} = 0.$$

But $x_2'(0) = x_1(0) = 1$.

We, thus, arrive at a contradiction, which means that $p^* > 0$. Here p^* is the smallest period. Historically, the number p^* has gained wide importance in trigonometry and its applications. Let us follow the convention in denoting the number p^* as 2π. The letter π was first used in this sense by William Jones in the year 1706 CE.

16.5 Some Particular Values

We have now obtained the period p^* of the functions $x_1(t)$ and $x_2(t)$. This number will help us find some intermediate values of $x_1(t)$ and $x_2(t)$. We have also obtained a number t^* such that $x_1(t^*) = 0$. For $t = 0$, we have $x_1(0) = 1$ and $x_2(0) = 0$. Since $x_1(t^*) = 0$, $x_2^2(t^*) = 1$

or $x_2(t^*) = \pm 1$. Since $x_1(t) > 0$ on $0 \le t < t^*$, in view of (2), $x_2(t)$ is an increasing function. With $x_2(0) = 0$, we can show that $x_1(2t^*) = -1$, $x_2(2t^*) = 0$, $x_1(3t^*) = 0$, $x_2(3t^*) = -1$, $x_1(4t^*) = 1$, $x_2(4t^*) = 0$.

We can state these values in the form of a table.

	$t = 0$	$t = t^*$	$t = 2t^*$	$t = 3t^*$	$t = 4t^* = 2\pi$
$x_1(t)$	1	0	-1	0	1
$x_2(t)$	0	1	0	-1	0

Further,

$$x_1(t^*) = 2x_1^2\left(\frac{t^*}{2}\right) - 1 = 0. \text{ Hence } x_1\left(\frac{t^*}{2}\right) = \frac{1}{\sqrt{2}} \text{ and}$$

$$x_2\left(\frac{t^*}{2}\right) = \frac{1}{\sqrt{2}}.$$

Using the relation

$$x_1(t^*) = 4x_1^3\left(\frac{t^*}{3}\right) - 3x_1\left(\frac{t^*}{3}\right) = 0,$$

we get

$$x_1\left(\frac{t^*}{3}\right)\left[4x_1^2\left(\frac{t^*}{3}\right) - 3\right] = 0. \text{ Since } x_1\left(\frac{t^*}{3}\right) \neq 0, \text{ we have}$$

$$x_1^2\left(\frac{t^*}{3}\right) = \frac{3}{4} \text{ or } x_1\left(\frac{t^*}{3}\right) = \pm\frac{\sqrt{3}}{2}.$$

We can at this stage obtain many values of $x_1(t)$ and $x_2(t)$ for particular choices of $t \in R$.

16.6 Other Trigonometrical Ratios

The functions $x_1(t)$ and $x_2(t)$ give rise to some additional functions whose properties can be derived from those obtained in our earlier discussion. These functions, defined below, also possess a period.

Define for $t \in R$, whenever these functions exist,

i. $z(t) = \dfrac{x_2(t)}{x_1(t)}$, $\qquad -\infty < z(t)\infty;$

ii. $w(t) = \dfrac{x_1(t)}{x_2(t)}$, $\qquad -\infty < w(t)\infty;$

iii. $p(t) = \dfrac{1}{x_2(t)}$, $\qquad -\infty < p(t) \le -1; \qquad 1 \le p(t) < \infty;$

iv. $q(t) = \dfrac{1}{x_1(t)}, \qquad -\infty < p(t) \leq -1; \qquad 1 \leq q(t) < \infty.$

The functions $z(t), w(t), p(t)$ and $q(t)$ are completely known in their interval of existence. By using the relations satisfied by $x_1(t)$ and $x_2(t)$, it is easy to derive the following relations,

a. $1 + z^2(t) = q^2(t)$,

b. $1 + w^2(t) = p^2(t)$,

c. $z(t)w(t) = 1$.

All the six functions x_1, x_2, z, w, p and q are called trigonometric functions and all the relations satisfied by these functions are called trigonometric formulae.

We have started the study of trigonometry by using the initial value problem (2). One can begin the study of trigonometry by using the system of equations

$$z' = q^2, \; q' = zq \tag{13}$$

with initial conditions $z(0) = 0, \; q(0) = 1$.

We can prove that for arbitrary $\alpha \in R$,

$$z(t+\alpha) = \frac{z(t) + z(\alpha)}{1 - z(t)z(\alpha)}$$

$$q(t+\alpha) = \frac{q(t)q(\alpha)}{1 - z(t)z(\alpha)}$$

Here we use the same technique as adopted in Section 15.3. We leave this proof to the readers. Through the functions z and q, we can define function $x_1(t)$ and $x_2(t)$ and establish their properties. The differential equations satisfied by $w(t)$ and $p(t)$ can also be a starting point. There details can be a project problem for students.

16.7 Infinite Series Solutions

Quite often it is convenient to obtain solutions $x_1(t)$, $x_2(t)$, of (2) and (3) in the form of infinite series. For this purpose, for $t \in R$ let,

$$x_1(t) = \sum_{n=0}^{\infty} b_n t^n \text{ and } \quad x_2(t) = \sum_{n=0}^{\infty} a_n t^n, \; -\infty < t < \infty \tag{14}$$

satisfy the equations (2) with initial conditions (3). Here $b_n, \; a_n, \; n = 0, 1, 2, \ldots$ are constants to be determined. Differentiate $x_1(t)$ and $x_2(t)$ term by term and substitute the values in (2). Compare the coefficients on either side and use initial data (3). This procedure gives us recurrence relations in terms of a_n and b_n. With the initial data at hand, we finally get the values of a_n and b_n, $n = 1, 2, 3 \ldots$. The conclusion is

$$x_1(t) = 1 - \frac{t^2}{2!} + \frac{t^4}{4!} - \frac{t^6}{6!} + \ldots = \sum_{n=0}^{\infty} (-1)^n \frac{t^{2n}}{(2n)!},$$

$$x_2(t) = t - \frac{t^3}{3!} + \frac{t^5}{5!} - \frac{t^7}{7!} + \ldots = \sum_{n=0}^{\infty} (-1)^n \frac{t^{2n+1}}{(2n+1)!}; \tag{15}$$

for $t \in R$.

Following similar techniques, we can obtain the infinite series solutions of (13) by using the series in (14) and finally obtain

$$z(t) = t + \frac{t^3}{3} + \frac{2t^5}{15} + \frac{17t^7}{315} + \frac{62t^9}{2835} + \cdots$$

and

$$q(t) = 1 + \frac{t^2}{2!} + \frac{5t^4}{4!} + \frac{6t^6}{6!} + \frac{1385t^8}{8!} + \ldots.$$

for $t \in R$. Series of this type have been widely employed in exploring the properties of trigonometric functions and their applications.

16.8 Zeros of solutions $x_1(t)$ and $x_2(t)$

The system $x_1' = -x_2,\ x_2' = x_1$ has a solution pair $(x_1(t), x_2(t))$ which is linearly independent.

By a zero of $x_1(t)$, we mean a value of t for which $x_1(t) = 0$. We have already established that solutions x_1 and x_2 possess infinite number of zeros. It will now be shown that the zeros of x_1 and x_2 interlace each other, i.e, between any two zeros of $x_1(t)$, there exists one and only one zero of $x_2(t)$ for $t \in R$.

Let t_1 and t_2 by any two consecutive zeros of $x_2(t)$, i.e $x_2(t_1) = x_2(t_2) = 0$. By the mean value theorem, there exists a number η, $t_1 < \eta < t_2$ such that $x_2'(\eta) = 0$, i.e $x_1(\eta) = 0$ in view of (2). Here η is a unique point, for, suppose there are points t_3 and $t_4, t_1 < t_3 < t_4 < t_2$ such that $x_1(t_3) = 0,\ x_1(t_4) = 0$. Then by the mean value property there is $\eta,\ t_1 < \eta < t_2$ such that $x_1'(\eta) = 0$. By(2) this means that $x_2(\eta) = 0$. This fact contradicts the assumption that t_1 and t_2 are two consecutive zeros of $x_2(t)$. Hence η is the only zero between t_1 and t_2 of $x_1(t)$.

If we draw the graphs of $x_1(t)$ and $x_2(t)$, we can easily observe the interlacing property of $x_1(t)$ and $x_2(t)$ for $t \epsilon R$.

16.9 Hyperbolic Functions

We have so far seen that trigonometrical functions are essentially the solutions of the system of differential equations (2) and (3). Most of the analytical properties of such functions are the trigonometrical formulae which we study by using traditional methods from our elementary course. It is natural to think about a related equation.

$$y'' - y = 0; \qquad y(0) = 1; \qquad y'(0) = 0. \tag{16}$$

This equation, as before, can be written in the form of a system of equations, equivalent to (2) and (3) by writing $y = y_1$ and

$$y_1^1 = y_2; \quad y_2^1 = y_1; \quad y_1(0) = 1; \quad y_2(0) = 0. \tag{17}$$

Let $(y_1(t), y_2(t))$ denote a solution pair of (17) for $t \in R$. Again note that equation (16) is linear, homogeneous, of second-order with constant coefficients and possess a unique solution. Clearly

$$y_1(t)y_1'(t) - y_2(t)y_2'(t) = y_1(t)y_2(t) - y_1(t)y_2(t) = 0.$$

On integration between 0 and t, we get $y_1^2(t) - y_2^2(t) = c$, (c is a constant of integration).

For $\quad t = 0, y_1^2(0) = 1$ and $y_2^2(0) = 0$. Hence $c = 1$.

We then get the first relation between $y_1(t)$ and $y_2(t)$, namely

$$y_1^2(t) - y_2^2(t) = 1. \tag{18}$$

Let $\alpha \in R$ be arbitrary. By following the argument in Section 15.3, we have the following addition formulae with respect to functions $y_1(t)$ and $y_2(t)$:

$$y_1(t+\alpha) = y_1(t)y_1(\alpha) + y_2(t)y_2(\alpha);$$

$$y_2(t+\alpha) = y_2(t)y_1(\alpha) + y_2(\alpha)y_1(t).$$

Further,

$$y_1(t-\alpha) = y_1(t)y_1(\alpha) - y_2(t)y_2(\alpha);$$

$$y_2(t-\alpha) = y_2(t)y_1(\alpha) - y_2(\alpha)y_1(t), t \in R.$$

For $\alpha = t$, we then have

$$y_1(2t) = y_1^2(t) + y_2^2(t); y_2(2t) = 2y_1(t)y_2(t).$$

These solutions $y_1(t)$ and $y_2(t)$ are called hyperbolic functions. They play as important a role in mathematics as the trigonometric functions $x_1(t)$ and $x_2(t) t \in R$.

It is obvious that we can define new functions $\frac{y_1(t)}{y_2(t)}, \frac{y_2(t)}{y_1(t)}, \frac{1}{y_1(t)}, \frac{1}{y_2(t)}$ and establish their properties. In order to be brief we leave this work as an exercise.

16.10 Nature of Wronskian Function

We have so far studied the differential equations (2),(3) and (17). The basic relations

$$x_1^2(t) + x_2^2(t) = 1,$$
$$y_1^2(t) - y_2^2(t) = 1;$$

given in (4) and (18) can be viewed from a different perspective. For the equations $x'' + x = 0,\ y'' - y = 0$, we can write the Wronskian property, namely,

$$W(x_1, x_2)(t) = \begin{vmatrix} x_1(t) & x_2(t) \\ -x_2(t) & x_1(t) \end{vmatrix} = e^{0.t} = 1$$

(0 is the coefficient of x' in the above equations);

similarly

$$W(y_1, y_2)(t) = \begin{vmatrix} y_1(t) & y_2(t) \\ y_1'(t) & y_2'(t) \end{vmatrix} = \begin{vmatrix} y_1(t) & y_2(t) \\ y_2(t) & y_1(t) \end{vmatrix} = e^{0.t} = 1.$$

The above relations suggests that a Wronskian function has close relations with the trigonometric and hyperbolic functions.

16.11 De Moivre's Result

We now relate solutions $x_1(t)$ and $x_2(t)$ to the exponential functions. Consider

$$e^{it} = 1 + it + \frac{(it)^2}{2!} + \frac{(it)^3}{3!} + \frac{(it)^4}{4!} + \ldots = \sum_{n=0}^{\infty} \frac{(it)^n}{n!} e^{it}$$

$$= \left(1 - \frac{t^2}{2!} + \frac{t^4}{4!} - \ldots\right) + i\left(t - \frac{t^3}{3!} + \frac{t^5}{5!} - \ldots\right)$$

$$= x_1(t) + ix_2(t).$$

Here we use the fact that $i = \sqrt{-1}$, $i^2 = -1$, and relations (15). Essentially, the infinite series representing $x_1(t)$ and $x_2(t)$ are two bisected sub-series of the exponential infinite series.

There are several interesting consequences of this result. For example,

$$e^{(int)} = (e^{it})^n = [x_1(t) + ix_2(t)]^n$$

$$= e^{i(nt)}$$

$$= x_1(nt) + ix_2(nt). \qquad (n \text{ is a rational number})$$

This is the well-known De Moivre's theorem. There are several applications of this result in literature.

Conclusion

The aim of this lecture was not to derive all trigonometrical and hyperbolic functions or obtain their properties and provide applications. The few sections written above provide a clue for an alternative method to study such functions which are widely used in mathematics. This alternative method is derived from the theory of differential equations and uses analytical methods to study the properties of solutions. The conclusion is that differential equations become a handy tool in studying many important functions. Refer to [1,3,4,5,9].

Another point that needs to be mentioned here is that the above sections are not the end of the story. In fact, it is to be remarked that this is the beginning of new directions in the development of trigonometrical and hyperbolic functions. For this purpose, we need to proceed to the next chapter " A Highway to Trigonometry II ".

Lecture 17

A Highway to Trigonometry II

Abstract
The present lecture aims at establishing extended trigonometric or trigonometric-like functions by considering higher order differentials. The methods used here are similar to those already considered in Lecture 16. We will also show that these methods help us establish matrix trigonometric and trigonometric-like functions. These ideas include the study of extended hyperbolic-like functions.

17.1 Introduction

In the last chapter, we started with linear, second order, homogeneous, initial value problems, $x'' \pm x = 0,\ x(0) = 1,\ x'(0) = 0$, and received a good dividend in the form of trigonometric and hyperbolic functions along with some of their properties. We also noted the elegance and simplicity of the alternative approach. It is indeed natural to investigate if higher order differential equations such as $x^{(n)} \pm x = 0$ with suitable initial conditions lead us to some new path. The answer to this enquiry is really positive. We do get solutions of such equations which are related to exponential functions and which share some of the properties of trigonometric-hyperbolic functions established earlier. In this lecture we will try to bring forth all such details. The immensity of the topic at hand reduces us to be brief in our presentation but we hope to give the reader a feel of the rewarding conclusions. For simplicity, we will describe the extensions for $n = 3$ in more detail.

17.2 Third Order Differential Equation

Consider a third order, linear, homogeneous differential equation:

$$x''' + x = 0, (' = d/dt), \quad t \in R, \tag{1}$$

with initial conditions

$$x(0) = 1, x'(0) = 0, x''(0) = 0. \tag{2}$$

This equation can be converted into a system of equations by writing $x = x_1$ and

$$x_1' = -x_3, \quad x_2' = x_1, \quad x_3' = x_2,$$

with initial conditions

$$x_1(0) = 1, \quad x_2(0) = 0 \;\; x_3(0) = 0. \tag{3}$$

The solution set $(x_1(t), x_2(t), x_3(t))$ of the system (3) exists on R uniquely. As in the previous lecture, we do not find the explicit solution set but will study the above triplet analytically. We multiply the first equation of (3) by $x_1^2 + x_2x_3$, the second equation by $-(x_2^2 - x_1x_3)$ and the third equation by $(x_3^2 + x_1x_2)$ and we find that

$$(x_1^2 + x_2x_3)x_1' - (x_2^2 - x_1x_3)x_2' + (x_3^2 + x_1x_2)x_3' = 0.$$

This relation can be verified from (3). The multiplication factors suggested here are by intuition only. The above relation can be written as

$$(x_1^2x_1' - x_2^2x_2' + x_3^2x_3') + (x_2x_3x_1' + x_1x_3x_2' + x_1x_2x_3') = 0.$$

Integration between 0 and t yields

$$\frac{x_1^3}{3} - \frac{x_2^3}{3} + \frac{x_3^3}{3} + x_1x_2x_3 = c; \text{ (c is a constant of integration).}$$

We rewrite this relation as

$$x_1^3(t) - x_2^3(t) + x_3^3(t) + 3x_1(t)x_2(t)x_3(t) = 3c$$

and determine c by using the initial data in (3).

For $t = 0$, we get

$$1 = 3c \text{ or } \quad c = 1/3. \text{ Hence}$$

$$x_1^3(t) - x_2^3(t) + x_3^3(t) + 3x_1(t)x_2(t)x_3(t) = 1; \quad t \in R. \tag{4}$$

This relation represents a surface in a 3-dimensional space. We can conclude that for each $t \in R$, the solution set $(x_1(t), x_2(t), x_3(t))$ generates a surface given in (4).

17.3 Wronskian Function

We employ an alternative method, the Wronskian function, to obtain the same relation. Here

$$W(x_1, x_2, x_3)(t) = \begin{vmatrix} x_1 & x_2 & x_3 \\ -x_3 & x_1 & x_2 \\ -x_2 & -x_3 & x_1 \end{vmatrix}(t) = W(0)e^{0t} = 1. \tag{5}$$

Here we have used the Wronskian property and noted that 0 is the coefficient of the term x'' in the equation $x''' + x = 0$. Now resolve the determinant to get

$$W(x_1, x_2, x_3) = x_1^3 - x_2^3 + x_3^3 + 3x_1x_2x_3 = 1, t \in R,$$

which is the same as (4).

Observe that in the earlier lecture we established the relation $x_1^2(t) + x_2^2(t) = 1$. The relation (4) now obtained can be considered as its extension in the third dimension, like a big brother. It is natural to expect that each equation of the family $x^{(n)} \pm x = 0$, $n = 4, 5, 6...$, has a similar formula which in a sense forms a family. Following a similar technique, readers may try to find the next big brother for $n = 4$ i.e., $x^{(4)} + x = 0$.

One can study the Wronskians in the previous lecture and the relation (5) above and observe the occurrence of the elements in the determinants. We then can conclude that the placement of elements is anti-circular. Determinants (matrices) of this type have interesting properties explored in literature. They also have many applications in engineering problems.

17.4 Infinite Series Solutions

We now consider the system (3) and obtain an infinite series solution, i.e., find an infinite series representing $x_1(t), x_2(t)$ and $x_3(t)$ for $t \in R$. For this purpose assume that

$$x_1(t) = \sum_{n=0}^{\infty} a_n t^n, x_2(t) = \sum_{n=0}^{\infty} b_n t^n, x_3(t) = \sum_{n=0}^{\infty} c_n t^n.$$

Now differentiate $x_1(t), x_2(t)$ and $x_3(t)$ term by term and substitute the values in (3) on both sides. Compare the coefficients of the same powers of t. This exercise will yield recurrence relations between the coefficient a_n, b_n, and c_n, $n = 0, 1, 2, ...$ Using the initial data in (3), we can get the values of the coefficient a_n, b_n and c_n for $n = 1, 2, 3....$ The long exercise will then yield the solutions

$$x_1(t) = 1 - \frac{t^3}{3!} + \frac{t^6}{6!} - \frac{t^9}{9!} + ... = \sum_{n=0}^{\infty}(-1)^n \frac{t^{3n}}{(3n)!};$$

$$x_2(t) = t - \frac{t^4}{4!} + \frac{t^7}{7!} - \frac{t^{10}}{10!} + ... = \sum_{n=0}^{\infty}(-1)^n \frac{t^{3n+1}}{(3n+1)!}; \tag{6}$$

$$x_3(t) = \frac{t^2}{2!} - \frac{t^5}{5!} + \frac{t^8}{8!} - \frac{t^{11}}{11!} + ... = \sum_{n=0}^{\infty}(-1)^n \frac{t^{3n+2}}{(3n+2)!};$$

for $t \in R$. It is indeed interesting to verify if x_1, x_2, x_3 in (6) are solutions of (3). Further, we ask the readers to compare the infinite series in (6) to those infinite series obtained in (15) of the earlier lecture.

17.5 Generalised Notation

The occurrence of various terms in (6) above suggests that we can introduce a more general notation which would aid in generalisation of the results for n. Define a function

$$M_{rj} = \sum_{n=0}^{\infty}(-1)^n \frac{t^{nr+j}}{(nr+j)!} \quad \begin{cases} r = 1, 2, 3\ldots, \infty \\ j = 0, 1, \ldots, r-1 \end{cases} \quad t \in R;$$

$$= \frac{t^j}{j!} - \frac{t^{r+j}}{(r+j)!} + \frac{t^{2r+j}}{(2r+j)!} - \frac{t^{3r+j}}{(3r+j)!} + \ldots \tag{7}$$

The notation $M_{r,j}$ simultaneously represent r infinite series, namely for a fixed r, $j = 0, 1, 2 \ldots r-1$,

i.e., $M_{r,1}(t), M_{r,2}(t), M_{r,3}(t), ...M_{r,r-1}(t)$. Here

$$M_{r,0}(t) = \sum_{n=0}^{\infty}(-1)^n \frac{t^{nr}}{(nr)!};$$

$$M_{r,1}(t) = \sum_{n=0}^{\infty}(-1)^n \frac{t^{nr+1}}{(nr+1)!};$$

$$M_{r,2}(t) = \sum_{n=0}^{\infty}(-1)^n \frac{t^{nr+2}}{(nr+1)!}; \text{ for } t \in R$$

and $$M_{r,r-1}(t) = \sum_{n=0}^{\infty}(-1)^n \frac{t^{(nr+r-1)}}{(nr+r-1)!}; \text{ for } t \in R.$$

Let us work out some particular infinite series (7):

i. let $r = 1, j = 0; M_{1,0} = \sum_{n=0}^{\infty} \frac{(-1)^n t^n}{(n)!} = e$

ii. let $r = 2, j = 0; M_{2,0}(t) = \sum_{n=0}^{\infty} \frac{(-1)^n t^{2n}}{(2n)!}$,

and for $r = 2, j = 1$,

$$M_{21}(t) = \sum_{n=0}^{\infty} (-1)^n \frac{t^{2n+1}}{(2n+1)!}.$$

Observe that these are the series $x_1(t)$ and $x_2(t)$ given by (15) in the previous lecture.

iii. $r = 3, j = 0, 1, 2, M_{3,0}(t) = \sum_{n=0}^{\infty} (-1)^n \frac{t^{3n}}{(3n)!}$;

$$M_{3,1}(t) = \sum_{n=0}^{\infty} (-1)^n \frac{t^{3n+1}}{(3n+1)!};$$

$$M_{3,2}(t) = \sum_{n=0}^{\infty} (-1)^n \frac{t^{3n+2}}{(3n+2)!}. \qquad (8)$$

Note that these are the series $x_1(t), x_2(t), x_3(t)$ given in (6). Clearly

$$M'''_{3,0}(t) + M_{3,0}(t) = 0; M_{3,0}(0) = 1, M'_{3,0}(0) = 0. M''_{3,0}(0) = 0;$$

$$M'''_{3,1}(t) + M_{3,1}(t) = 0; M_{3,1}(0) = 0, M'_{3,1}(0) = 1. M''_{3,1}(0) = 0;$$

$$M'''_{3,2}(t) + M_{3,2}(t) = 0; M_{3,2}(0) = 0, M'_{3,2}(0) = 0. M''_{3,2}(0) = 0.$$

Further, the relation (5) now takes the form

$$W(x_1, x_2, x_3)(t) = W(M_{3,0}, M_{3,1}, M_{3,2})(t)$$

$$= \begin{vmatrix} M_{3,0}(t) & M_{3,1}(t) & M_{3,2}(t) \\ -M_{3,2}(t) & M_{3,0}(t), & M_{3,1}(t) \\ -M_{3,1}(t), & -M_{3,2}(t), & M_{3,0}(t) \end{vmatrix}$$

$$= M^3_{3,0}(t) - M^3_{3,1}(t) + M^3_{3,2}(t) + 3M_{3,0}M_{3,1}M_{3,2}.$$

We present in Figs. 17.1–17.4 the nature of graphs of the trigonometric-like functions given in (6) and (4).

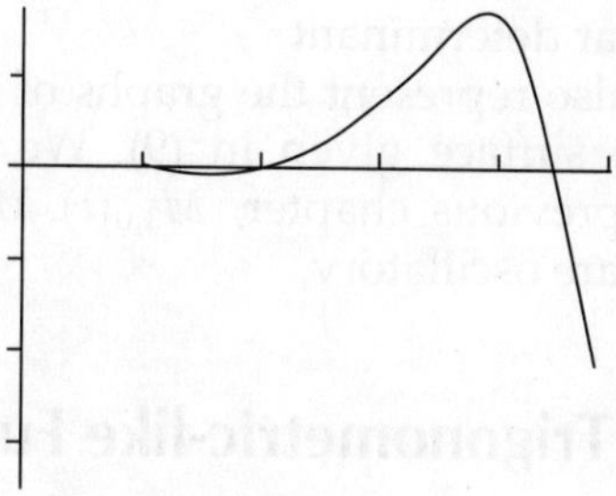

Fig. 17.1 Graph of $M_{3.0}(t)$

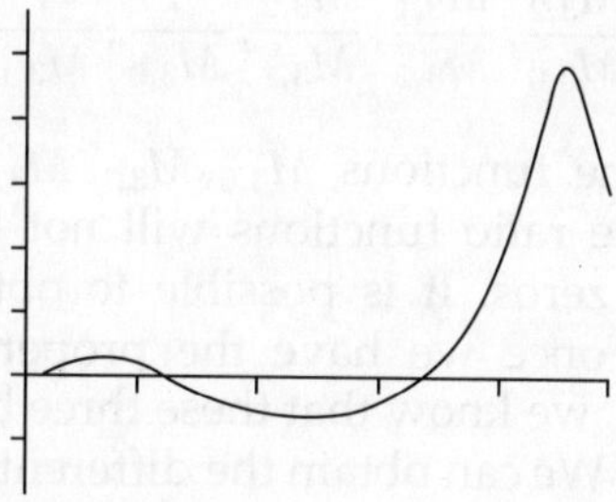

Fig. 17.2 Graph of $M_{3.1}(t)$

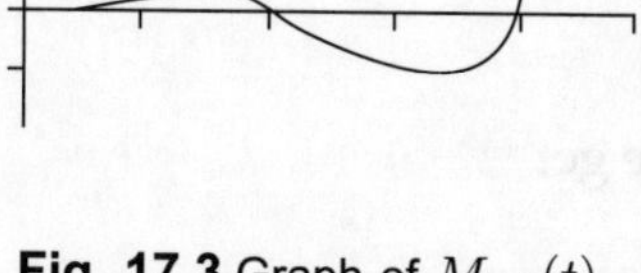

Fig. 17.3 Graph of $M_{3.2}(t)$

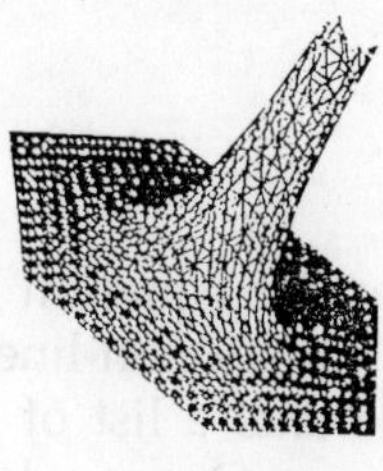

Fig. 17.4 Graph of $M_{3.0}^3 - m_{3.1}^3 + M_{3.2}^3 + 3M_{3.0}M_{3.1}M_{3.2} = 1$ (9)

This is an anti-circular determinant.

The Figs 17.1–17.4 also represent the graphs of the functions $M_{3,0}(t)$, $M_{3,1}(t)M_{3,2}(t)$ and the surface given in (9). We observe that, unlike $M_{2,0}(t), M_{2.,}(t)$ of the previous chapter, $M_{3,0}(t), M_{3,1}(t), M_{3,2}(t)$ are not periodic functions but are oscillatory.

17.6 Additional Trigonometric-like Functions

Having defined $M_{3,0}$, $M_{3,1}$ and $M_{3,2}$, we can define additional trigonometric-like functions by considering the ratios of these functions. These are

$$\frac{M_{3,0}}{M_{3,1}}, \frac{M_{3,0}}{M_{3,2}}, \frac{M_{3,1}}{M_{3,0}}, \frac{M_{3,2}}{M_{3,0}}, \frac{M_{3,1}}{M_{3,2}}, \frac{M_{3,2}}{M_{3,1}}, \frac{1}{M_{3,0}}, \frac{1}{M_{3,1}}, \frac{1}{M_{3,2}},$$

for $t \in R$. Note that the functions $M_{3,0}, M_{3,1}, M_{3,2}$ are oscillatory and have infinite zeros. The ratio functions will not be defined when the denominators become zeros. It is possible to obtain many properties of the ratio functions once we have the properties of the functions $M_{3.0}, M_{3.1}, M_{3.2}$ at hand, we know that these three basic functions are the solutions of $x''' + x = 0$. We can obtain the differential equations satisfied by the ratio functions.

Let us try to obtain the differential equations satisfied by $M_{3,0}/M_{3,1}$.

Let $y(t) = \dfrac{M_{3,0}(t)}{M_{3,1}(t)}$. Differentiate y and use the fact that,

$$M'_{3,0}(t) = -M_{3,2}(t), M'_{3,1}(t) = M_{3,0}(t) \text{ and } M'_{3,2}(t) = M_{3,1}(t)$$

to get

$$y' + y^2 = \frac{-M_{3,2}}{M_{3,1}}.$$

Differentiating again we get

$$y'' + 2yy' = -1\frac{-M_{3,2}}{M_{3,1}}y = -1 + (-y' - y_2)y.$$

Hence we get

$$y'' + 3yy' + y^3 + 1 = 0.$$

This is a non-linear second order equation having solution $M_{3,0}/M_{3,1}$. In general all ratio functions satisfy non-linear differential equations of higher orders. Table 17.1 presents a list of such differential equations along with their explicit solutions. Once we know their explicit solutions, we can derive their properties. One may also consider $f(M_{3,0}, M_{3,1}, M_{3,2})$

to obtain additional non-linear differential equations. Observe that we have done this excercise for only $n = 3$. A similar exercise can be done for $n = 4, 5, 6 \ldots$. Obviously the task will be difficult.

Differential equation	solution(s)
$y'' + 3yy' + y^3 + 1 = 0$	$\frac{M_{3,0}}{M_{3,1}}$
$y'' + 3yy' - y^3 + 1 = 0$	$\frac{M_{3,1}}{M_{3,2}}$
$y'' - 3yy' + y^3 - 1 = 0$	$\frac{M_{3,2}}{M_{3,0}}$
$y''y - 2y'^2 + 3y' - y^3 - 1 = 0$	$\frac{M_{3,0}}{M_{3,2}}$
$y''y - 2y]^2 + 3y' - y^3 - 1 = 0$	$\frac{M_{3,1}}{M_{3,0}}$
$y''y - 2y'^2 + 3y' - y^3 - 1 = 0$	$\frac{M_{3,2}}{M_{3,1}}$
$y''' + 3y'' + 3y' + 2y = 0$	$e^{-z}M_{3,1}$
$y''' + 4yy'' + 6y^2y'' + 3y'^2 + y^4 + 1 = 0$	$\frac{M_{4,0}}{M_{4,1}}$
$y'' + 4yy'' + 6y^2y'' + 3y'^2 + y^4 + 1 = 0$	$\frac{M_{4,1}}{M_{4,2}}$
$y''' + 2yy'' + 3y'^2 - y^4 + 1 = 0$	$\frac{M_{4,2}}{M_{4,3}}$
$y''' - 2yy'' - 3y'^2 + y^4 - 1 = 0$	$\frac{M_{4,3}}{M_{4,0}}$

Table 17.1 Differential equations and their solutions

17.7 Additional Formulae

In (5), (6) and (10) of Lecture 16, Section 16.3, we have proved the "addition formulae" for solutions $(x_1(t), x_2(t))$ i.e., $M_{2,0}(t), M_{2,1}(t)$. The question that immediately enters our mind is whether similar formulae exist for solutions $y_1(t), y_2(t)$ and $y_3(t)$ i.e. $M_{3,0}(t), M_{3,1}(t), M_{3,2}(t)$ for $t \in R$. The answer to this query is 'yes', such addition formulae do exist. Let us follow the same procedure we used in Lecture 16.

We know that $M_{3,0}(t), M_{3,1}(t), M_{3,2}(t)$ are three linearly independent solutions of (1) or the equivalent system (3). Let $\alpha \in R$ be arbitrary. Clearly $M_{3,0}(t+\alpha), M_{3,1}(t+\alpha), M_{3,2}(t+\alpha)$ are also solutions of (1) and

$$M_{3,0}(t+\alpha) = c_1 M_{3,0}(t) + C_2 M_{3,1}(t) + C_2 M_{3,2}(t), t \in R, \alpha \in R \qquad (10)$$

Here c_1, c_2, c_3 are constants (they depend on α) to be determined. For $t = 0$, we have,

$$M_{3,0}(\alpha) = c_1 M_{3,0}(0) + c_2 M_{3,1}(0) + c_3 M_{3,2}(0) = c_1.$$

Here we have to recall the initial data given in (3). Thus, we have obtained the value of c_1. Now differentiate (10) to get

$$M'_{3,0}(t+\alpha) = c_1 M'_{3,0}(t) + c_2 M'_{3,1}(t) + c_3 M'_{3,2}(t)$$

i.e., $-M_{3,2}(t+\alpha) = -c_1 M_{3,2}(t) + c_2 M_{3,0}(t) + c_3 M_{3,1}(t).$ (11)

At $t = 0$, we get

$$-M_{3,2}(\alpha) = -c_1 M_{3,2}(0) + c_2 M_{3,0}(0) + c_3 M_{3,1}(0) = c_2.$$

We now differentiate (11) to get

$$-M'_{3,2}(t+\alpha) = c_1 M'_{3,2}(t) + c_2 M'_{3,0}(t) + c_3 M'_{3,2}(t);$$

$$-M_{3,1}(t+\alpha) = -c_1 M_{3,1}(t) - c_2 M_{3,2}(t) + c_3 M_{3,1}(t).$$

At $t = 0$, we have

$$-M_{3,1}(\alpha) = -c_1 M_{3,1}(0) - c_2 M_{3,2}(0) + c_3 M_{3,0}(0) = c_3.$$

Thus, we have successfully obtained the values of c_1, c_2 and c_3. Substituting these values in (10), we obtain the addition formulae for $M_{3,0}(t)$ given by

$$M_{3,0}(t+\alpha) = M_{3,0}(t)M_{3,0}(\alpha) - M_{3.1}(t)M_{3,2}(\alpha) - M_{3,2}(t)M_{3,1}(\alpha).$$

By following a similar procedure, we prove that

$$M_{3,1}(t+\alpha) = M_{3,0}(t)M_{3,1}(\alpha) + M_{3,1}(t)M_{3,0}(\alpha) - M_{3,2}(t)M_{3,2}(\alpha)$$

and

$$M_{3,2}(t+\alpha) = M_{3,0}(t)M_{3,2}(\alpha) + M_{3,1}(t)M_{3,1}(\alpha) + M_{3,2}(t)M_{3,0}(\alpha);$$

$t \in R$. Thus we have three addition formulae at our disposal.

It is now easy to derive

$$M_{3,0}(2t) = M^2_{3,0}(t) - 2M_{3,1}(t)M_{3,2}(t);$$

$$M_{3,1}(2t) = 2M_{3,0}(t)M_{3,1}(t) - M^2_{3,2}(t);$$

$$M_{3,2}(2t) = 2M_{3,0}(t)M_{3,2}(t) + M^2_{3,1}(t).$$

We can also obtain $M_{3,0}(3t), M_{3,1}(3t), M_{3,2}(3t)$. Many similar extensions are possible.

The above technique has obvious extensions for functions $M_{r,j}(t+\alpha), j = 0, 1, 2, ...r-1$, and $r = 4, 5, 6, ...$

17.8 The Characteristic Equation

The characteristic equation of $x^{(r)} + x = 0$ is $z^r + 1 = 0$. When $r = 2$, we get $z^2 + 1 = 0$ having characteristic roots $z = \pm\, i$. In Lecture 16, Section 16.11, we exploited the properties of the complex number i. One of the queries can be: is there an equivalent development for the equation $x''' + x = 0$ having the characteristic equation, $z^3 + 1 = 0$? Do the solutions of this polynomial equation play similar roles as the roots of $z^2 + 1 = 0$? We attempt to answer these questions.

The cubic equation $z^3 + 1 = 0$ has the roots $-1, \dfrac{1-i\sqrt{3}}{2}, \dfrac{1+i\sqrt{3}}{2}$. Let us denote these roots by the notation $-1,\ w,\ -w^2$. Consider for $t \in R$,

$$e^{-t} = 1 - t + \frac{t^2}{2!} - \frac{t^3}{3!} + \frac{t^4}{4!} - \ldots$$

$$= (1 - \frac{t^3}{3!} + \frac{t^6}{6!} - \ldots) - (t - \frac{t^4}{4!} + \frac{t^7}{7!} - \ldots) + (\frac{t^2}{2!} - \frac{t^5}{5!} + \frac{t^8}{8!} \ldots)$$

$$= M_{3,0}(t) \ - M_{3,1}(t) + M_{3,2}(t). \tag{12}$$

Thus the series of e^{-t} is trisected and we express each part by a sub-series of e^{-t}. This is, in fact, what we did in the previous lecture. Similarly

$$e^{wt} = M_{3,0}(t) + wM_{3,1}(t) + w^2 M_{3,2}(t); \tag{13}$$

$$e^{-w^2 t} = M_{3,0}(t) - wM_{3,2}(t) - w^2 M_{3,1}(t). \tag{14}$$

Observe that since w is a root of $z^3 + 1 = 0$, $w^3 + 1 = 0$. We have used this fact to develop (13) and (14). There are several interesting consequences of the relations (12), (13) and (14) in which we have employed the sub-series $M_{3,0}$, $M_{3,1}$ and $M_{3,2}$. In (12), if we replace t by nt (n is a rational number), we have

$$e^{-nt} = M_{3,0}(nt) - M_{3,1}(nt) + M_{3,2}(nt), t \in R.$$

Further, from (13), we have

$$e^{wnt} = (e^{wt})^n$$

$$= [M_{3,0}(t) + wM_{3,1}(t) + w^2 M_{3,2}(t)]^n$$

$$= e^{w(nt)}$$

$$= M_{3,0}(nt) + wM_{2,1}(nt) + w^2 M_{3,2}(nt), t \in R.$$

Also,

$$(e^{-w^2 t})^n = e^{-w^2 nt}$$

$$= [M_{3,0}(t) - wM_{3,2}(t) - w^2 M_{3,1}(t)]^n$$

$$= e^{-w^2(nt)}$$

$$= M_{3,0}(nt) - wM_{3,2}(nt) - w^2 M_{3,1}(nt).$$

The three relations are the extensions of the well-known De Moivre's theroem. These results have not yet been applied else where.

17.9 Laplace Transforms

For several applications, we need Laplace transforms. Let us work out the L-transforms of $M_{3,0}, M_{3,1}, M_{3,2}$

$$L(M_{3,0}(t)) = \int_0^\infty e^{-st} M_{3,0}(t)dt$$

$$= \int_0^\infty e^{-st} \left[\sum_{n=0}^\infty (-1)^n \frac{t^{3n}}{(3n)!}\right] dt$$

$$= \sum_{n=0}^\infty \frac{(-1)^n}{(3n)!} \int_0^\infty e^{-st} t^{3n} dt$$

$$= \sum_{n=0}^\infty \frac{(-1)^n}{s^{n+1}} = \frac{s^2}{s^3+1}.$$

Similarly, we can prove that

$$L(M_{3,1}(t)) = \frac{s}{s^3+1} \text{ and } L(M_{3,2}(t)) = \frac{1}{s^3+1}$$

$$L(M'_{3,0}(t)) = -M_{3,0}(0) + sL(M_{3,0}(t))$$

$$= -1 + s.\frac{s^2}{s^3+1}$$

$$= \frac{-1}{s^3+1}$$

$$= -L(M_{3,2}(t)).$$

Other relations can be similarly obtained. All such relations can be used in applications and for solving initial and boundary value problems of differential and integral equations. Students can attempt such problems in their project works.

17.10 A Project for Students

In order to develop the relations for extended hyperbolic functions, consider the differential equation.

$$x''' - x = 0,\ x(0) = 1,\ x'(0) = 0,\ x''(0) = 0, \quad t \in R$$

or its equivalent system of equations

$$x_1' = x_3, x_2' = x_1, x_3' = x_2, x(0) = 1, x'(0) = 0, x''(0) = 0.$$

1. Show that the infinite series
   $N_{3,0}(t) = \sum_{n=0}^{\infty} \frac{t^{3n}}{(3n)!}$, $N_{3,1}(t) = \sum_{n=0}^{\infty} \frac{t^{3n+1}}{(3n+1)!}$
   $N_{3,2}(t) = \sum_{n=0}^{\infty} \frac{t^{3n+2}}{(3n+2)!}$ are three linearly independent solutions of the system.

2. For $\alpha \in R$, a constant, find the relations for $N_{3,0}(t+\alpha)$,$N_{3,1}(t+\alpha)$ and $N_{3,2}(t+\alpha)$ and use these formulae to find $N_{3,0}(2t)$; $N_{3,1}(2t)$; $N_{3,2}(2t)$; $N_{3,0}(3t)$; $N_{3,1}(3t)$; $N_{3,2}(3t)$.

3. Show that
   $N_{3,0}^3(t) + N_{3,1}^3(t) + N_{3,2}^3(t) - 3N_{3,0}(t)N_{3,1}(t)N_{3,2}(t) = 1$,
   (use the Wronskian formula)

4. Find the roots of the characteristic equation $z^3 - 1 = 0$ and use these to establish De Moivre's theorem.

5. Find the Laplace transforms of $N_{3,0}(t), N_{3,1}(t), N_{3,2}(t)$.

6. Define the ratios
   $\frac{N_{3,0}}{N_{3,1}}, \frac{N_{3,1}}{N_{3,0}}, \frac{N_{3,1}}{N_{3,2}}, \frac{N_{3,2}}{N_{3,1}}, \frac{N_{3,2}}{N_{3,0}}, \frac{N_{3,0}}{N_{3,2}}, \frac{1}{N_{3,0}}, \frac{1}{N_{3,1}}, \frac{1}{N_{3,2}}$.
   Find the differential equations of which these ratios are solutions.

Conclusion

In the earlier sections of this lecture we obtained several results on extended trigonometric functions and hyperbolic functions. Readers will note that not every property that we come across in trigonometry is touched here. However, the given results will help us build additional properties. Students, while preparing for a project (refer to [3]), can establish the remaining results and obtain applications. One question that needs to be answered is: is it the end of the development of trigonometry and hyperbolic functions? The answer is certainly, "no".

One may consider matrices of order $n \times n$ and explore the development of e^{At}, where A is an $n \times n$ matrix. Many results in the matrix form of trigonometric and hyperbolic functions are known. Further, one may consider the space of linear bounded operators on abstract Banach spaces. Here we can extend the earlier results. It is of course necessary to create illustrative examples. We do not deal with these areas of literature here since it is beyond the intended scope of the book. Refer to [6, 7, 8, 10] for advanced work.

Lecture 18

Mathematical Theory of Collective Decisions

Abstract

Predicting the possible collective decision about various aspects of a single problem has interesting possibilities. In a country like India where democracy (rule by majority) governs all social, educational and political institutes, from villages to parliament, imagine how it would be if we could predict the collective decision made by the majority. Therefore, any theory relating to this problem has a wide scope for application in further mathematical and statistical studies. We will provide here an elementary introduction to a mathematical theory of collective decisions.

18.1 Introduction

The importance of a mathematical theory for collective decisions need not be overemphasised in a democratic set up, where the collective decision by the majority governs all social, educational and political institutions from villages to parliament. The main problem is to predict in advance the possible collective decision. Only an elementary introduction to this well-developed topic is presented here.

18.2 Median Rule

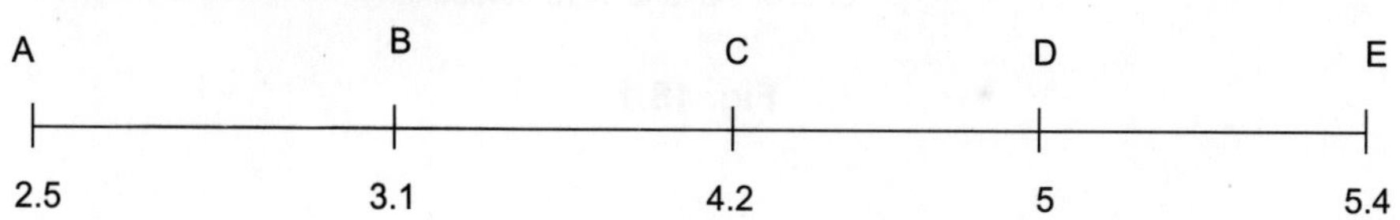

Suppose a committee of five persons A, B, C, D, E has been set up to finalise the budget for the construction of a school building. A believes that 2.5 lakhs is sufficient, while B wants a budget of 3.1 lakhs, C: 4.2 lakhs, D: 5 lakhs and E: 5.4 lakhs. A majority decision is required i.e., if three persons support a budget, it is sanctioned. Obviously a majority will support a budget of 4.2 lakhs, since the tendency of each person is to prefer a proposal closer to his opinion. Thus for example if 5 lakhs is proposed by D, it will be rejected by A, B, C, as 4.2 is closer to their choice than 5. Ultimately the decision will be a budget of 4.2 lakhs. This 4.2 is called an equilibrium point of the decision space: a point which is preferred over all other points by a simple majority.

18.3 Preferential Ranking

Suppose a farmer wants to buy a land. Although in reality, he must consider many aspects before taking a decision about it, for simplicity, we assume that he considers only two aspects: i) the cost of the available land and ii) its location measured by the distance of the land from his village home. Suppose his top priority is for minimum cost and the distance is of secondary importance. The preferred choice of the farmer and the available land are shown in the graph in Fig 18.1.

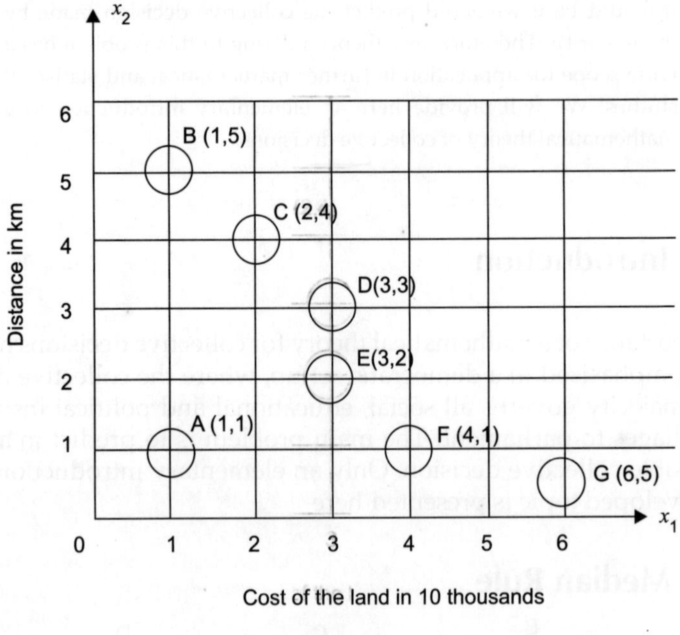

Fig. 18.1

The optimal option of the farmer is Rs. 10,000 and 1 km, which is shown by the point A. Other options available to him are shown by points B, C, D, E, F and G. There is no land available as per the farmer's, optimal choice. He must therefore decide his order of preference by choosing successively the available alternatives. He will thus rank his salience (preference) as follows by considering the cost first and the distance next: B C E D F G.

The points E and D are available at the same cost of Rs. 30,000/-. He then applies his second criteria and prefers E to D. A new criteria for measuring closeness is applied here. For example, B is closer to A than F according to this criteria though distance AF = 3 and distance AB = 4 and so AB > AF. Such an ordering of points on a plane is called lexicographic ordering. In this kind of ordering, we place the points in ascending order according to the first coordinate only. In case there is a tie between two points due to equality of the first coordinate, we resolve the tie by taking the point with the nearest second coordinate, first. If the farmer gave importance to distance, his preferences would be G F E D C B.

18.4 Majority Decision

Ignore the points A and G in Fig 18.1. Suppose B, C, D, E, F are members of a committee who wish to decide about the purchase of a land for the agricultural school run by them. For simplicity, suppose only two aspects are considered: 1) the budget to be sanctioned (x_1-axis) and 2) the allowable distance from the school (x_2-axis). All members unanimously agree that the issue of cost is more important than the distance. The opinions of the members are represented by the two coordinates. Thus for example B wants to stress that a budget of Rs. 10000 should be sanctioned and the distance 5 km can be allowed. Similarly each other member vehemently stresses the option given by the coordinates for him in the figure. What will be the final decision of the committee? Each member uses the principal of lexicographic ordering to rank his salience.

SOLUTION

The majority here is 3. Draw a straight line parallel to x_2-axis so that there are less than 3 individuals on either side of it. This is the straight line in the figure called the x_1-median. On this median, x_1 is constant = 3; and there are only two points (less than majority 3) on either side of the x_1-median DE. Similarly draw a straight line parallel to x_1-axis such that there are less than 3 individuals on either side of it. This line through D is called the x_2-median. The intersection of the two medians is then the decision point. A budget of Rs. 30000/- and a location up to 3 kms from school will be sanctioned in the meeting.

For, if any point to the left or right of the x_1-median is proposed, then it will be rejected by a simple majority on the right or left side respectively of

3 and 4 individuals. This is because there are better proposals preferable to them than these proposals. Hence the decision point must be on the x_1-median. Similarly it has to be on the x_2-median. Hence D is the desired decision point. It is also called an equilibrium point.

Equilibrium point: It is defined as a point in the policy space such that there is no other point which a simple majority prefers to this point. The solutions above gives a simple theorem.

THEOREM 1

When the committee has an odd number of members, and simple majority rule is being used, the intersection of the two median lines is the equilibrium point.

18.5 Even Number of Members

Let us take the same figure given in Fig. 18.1 and include the point G in it, so that there are now $m = 6$ members on the committee. What will be the probable decision of the committee?

SOLUTION

The majority number is now $K = 4$. Draw a straight line $x_1 = x_{1b}$ such that there are atmost $K - 1 = 4 - 1 = 3$ members to the left of it in the half plane $x_1 < x_{1b}$, and there are atmost $m - K = 6 - 4 = 2$ members to the right of it in the half plane $x_1 > x_{1b}$. This is the line DE in our figure given by $x_1 = x_{1b} = 3$ called the right x_1-median. Similarly draw a straight line $x_1 = x_{1a}$ such that there are almost $K - 1 = 3$ members to the right of it i.e., $x_1 > x_{1a}$, while there are almost $m - K = 2$ members to the left side $x_1 < x_{1a}$. This is called the left x_1-median. In the specific example given by our figure, the left and right medians coincide in the line DE with the equation $x_1 = 3$.

Similarly we can draw the upper and lower medians $x_2 = x_{2b} = 3$ through D and $x_2 = x_{2a} = 2$ through E. The decision will be on $x_1 = 3$ between D and E. There is an uncertainty in the decision as far as the distance from the school is concerned, though the budget of Rs. 30000 is agreed. Any proposal represented by a point outside the segment $\overline{\text{DE}}$ will be rejected by simple majority rule, and the proposal points will be moving inwards. But as soon as some one proposes an alternative represented by any point on $\overline{\text{DE}}$ for the first time, it will be unanimously agreed, as there is no simple majority to reject this proposal. Thus out of the many possible equilibrium points on $\overline{\text{DE}}$, the one proposed first will be the final decision of the committee.

In general, if $x_{1a} \neq x_{2a}$ and $x_{1b} \neq x_{2b}$, there will be a rectangle bounded by the four medians, and the point proposed first from the interior of this rectangle will represent the final decision.

THEOREM 2

The equilibrium set is the intersection of the four regions $x_1 \geq x_{1a}$, $x_1 \leq x_{1b}$, $x_2 \geq x_{2a}$, $x_2 \leq x_{2b}$.

18.6 Extension of the Results

Weighted opinions

We have taken a model in which no two members have the same opinion. If the committee consists of several groups, each holding a fixed opinion, then the mathematics does not change essentially. For example there may be $n = w_1 + w_2 + w_3 + w_4 + w_5$ members, out of which w_1 have the opinion A (1,5) etc. If n is odd the majority number is $(n+1)/2 = (w_1 + w_2 + w_3 + w_4 + w_5 + 1)/2$. Now we can have our two medians as before, their intersection giving the decision point, whose coordinates give the final decision. This is the case of five groups of members, with n odd. In case n is even, we will get a rectangular region, the interior of which consists of possible decision points as before.

Example: It may be verified by this procedure that if there are five groups with $w_1 = 2, w_2 = 3, w_3 = 3, w_4 = 2, w_5 = 5$, then $K = 8$ is the majority rule and D (3,3) indicating Rs. 30000/- for budget and a distance up to 3 kms is the decision point. If $w_1 = 11, w_2 = w_3 = w_4 = w_5 = 1$ then B (1,5) indicating a budget of Rs. 10000/- and a distance up to 5 kms is the decision point. The two medians pass through A.

18.7 Higher Dimensional Policy Space

There may be more than two criteria for the committee to consider with a need for the members to reach an unanimous agreement about their importance in order of preference. If there are n aspects under consideration, the policy space is now n-dimensional. Any option in this space can be represented by $x = (x_1, x_2 \ldots x_{n-1}, x_n)$. The $2n$ medians are now $(n-1)$ dimensional hyperplanes and the box-type region bounded by them is the decision region which will be a simple point if the total number of members is odd.

18.8 Different Salience Groups in the Same Committee

Consider again a two-dimensional policy space (cost and distance for example) and suppose one group of members give utmost importance to cost, while the distance is most important for the other group. The following theorem can be proved in this case

THEOREM 3

If a committee, all of whose members order the alternatives (x_1, x_2) of a two-dimensional policy space lexicographically, is composed of two different salience groups, then the equilibrium region under simple majority rule is the intersection of (i) the region bounded by group one's vertical median lines $x_1 = x_{1a}, x_1 = x_{1b}$ and group two's horizontal median lines $x_2 = x_{2g}, x_2 = x_{2h}$ and (ii) the region bounded by the four medians of the whole committee, if all used the same lexicographic ranking of the policy dimensions.

18.9 Preferences are not Numbers

If we consider for example, the set p of all political parties in India, then its elements are not numbers. But since a couple of allied parties may be closer to each other (in terms of ideology, policy etc.) than the rest, it may be possible to represent p as an ordered (not necessarily totally ordered) set. Similarly, each other attribute involved in an election may be represented by an ordered set. As before, we may assume the same preferential ranking of these attributes by voters. Then the output of voting (a collective decision) may be analysed as before and the final decision may be predicted, though we are not using numbers for ranking.

Conclusion

Predicting the results of collective decisions, including those in the general political elections, based on data, sample surveys and statistical or mathematical analysis, is now a complex problem of great importance. The elementary aspects of this problem discussed here are those presented by Michael Taylor in *Mathematical Approaches to Politics*. We hope it will initiate readers into further extensive and deeper studies.

Lecture 19

Satellite Dynamics

Abstract

The basic theory of central orbits, taught at the graduate level, is applied to solve a variety of important problems in satellite dynamics especially for the circular or elliptic paths taken by satellites.

19.1 Introduction

One of the several means of popularising mathematics is to emphasise its interesting applications to a variety of realistic important problems. Even an introductory course on mechanics, taught at the graduate level, can be fruitfully used for this purpose. A complex problem like discovering the dynamics of a sphere moving down a smooth inclined plane, which is itself sliding on a rough horizontal plane may be a good intellectual challenge for applying basic principles, but a student unable to visualise a real-life situation where such a complex problem may occur, may soon loose interest in the subject. Such so-called applied mathematics is as good as that pure mathematics, which is far away from applications. Unfortunately many textbooks on mechanics are full of such solved and unsolved complex unrealistic problems and they have contributed in making the subject unpopular and uninteresting in the graduate course itself. Therefore such problems should be replaced by some modern applications of mechanics.

Thinking over this matter, we felt that the following three current interesting problems of the 20th and 21st century can be introduced in dynamics to make it more alive.

1. Launching of a rocket for installing satellites, hitting targets, etc.
2. Satellite dynamics.
3. Pursuit curves: The paths travelled by guided missiles for hitting a moving or fixed target.

It is possible to introduce these problems via a simple model avoiding some ingredient complexities. Satellite dynamics is introduced here from this point of view. The other two topics will also appear in this book subsequently in Lecture 20 and 21.

19.2 The Problem and its Importance

The Moon is a natural satellite of the Earth, while all planets are satellites of the Sun. Copying this natural phenomenon, man-made satellites have been launched from the Earth's surface with the help of multistage rockets. They revolve round the centre, E of the Earth in periodic circular or elliptic orbits. They are used for many purposes, for example

i. Civil communications through Internet and TV programmes, military communications,
ii. Weather forecasting,
iii. Guiding ballistic missiles involving very long range projections.
iv. Data collection on other planets by launching satellites around them.
v. Intermediate space stations in the Universe.

19.3 Basic Theory

The theory used is the standard theory of central orbits, governed by Newton's laws of motion, explained in all textbooks. The following are also used.

19.3.1 Newton's Law of Gravitation

The force of attraction between any two particles of masses m_1 and m_2 is directly proportional to the product $m_1 m_2$ of the masses and inversely proportional to the square of the distance between them.

A brief outline of the theory as presented in the book, *Modern Introduction to Classical Mechanics, and Control*, by Burghes D N and Downs A M, is given here to make this article self-contained.

Let m, M be respectively the masses of the satellite and Earth, concentrated at their centroids S, E respectively. Then the attraction of the Earth in the direction $\overrightarrow{\text{SE}}$ on the satellites is of magnitude $F = \gamma mM/R^2, R = ES$, where γ is the gravitational constant whose value is $6.67 \times 10^{-11} \text{m}^3\,\text{kg}^{-1}\,\text{s}^2$; M = mass of the Earth = 5.976×10^{24} kg. According to Newton's second law of motion, this force along $\overrightarrow{\text{SE}}$ = (m. Acceleration of S along $\overline{\text{SE}}$). This is the basic equation of motion of the satellite S.

19.3.2 Satellite in a Circular Orbit

Let $R_E \cong 6368$ km be the radius of the Earth, while h is the constant height of the satellite above the Earth's surface, so that the constant radius R_0 of the circular orbit is ES $= R_E + h$ (Fig. 19.1). The magnitude of acceleration of S along SE in this case is v^2/R_0, where v is the speed of S. The force of attraction along $\overrightarrow{\text{SE}}$ is $\gamma mM/R_0$. Hence the equation of motion of S is

$$\frac{mv^2}{R_0} = \frac{\gamma mM}{R_0^2}$$

so that,

$$v^2 = \frac{K}{R_0} = \frac{K}{(R_E + h)^2}; \; K = \gamma M \tag{1}$$

This equation gives a relation between the constant height h of S above the Earth's surface and the constant velocity of S.

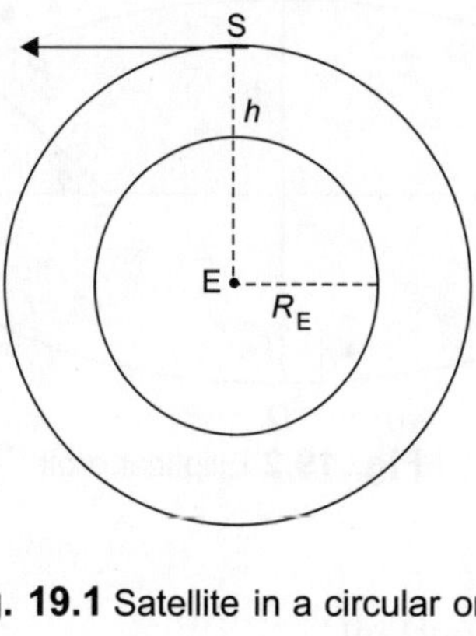

Fig. 19.1 Satellite in a circular orbit

19.3.3 Period of the Orbit

The time required by S to complete one revolution about the centre E is called the period of the orbit. Then the radius vector $\overrightarrow{ES}$ has an angular velocity $\omega = 2\pi/T$, which is the angle through which $\overrightarrow{ES}$ rotates per unit time. Thus the magnitude v of the velocity of S is

$$v = R_0\omega = (R_E + h)\frac{2\pi}{T}. \tag{2}$$

Substituting from (2) in (1), we have

$$T = \left(\frac{2\pi}{\sqrt{\gamma M}}\right) R_0^{3/2} = \left(\frac{2\pi}{\sqrt{K}}\right) R_0^{3/2}. \tag{3}$$

Thus T^2 is proportional to R_0^3 which is in accordance with Kepler's third law.

19.3.4 Non-circular Orbits

In this case (Fig. 19.2), the acceleration of S has a radial component $\ddot{R} - R\dot{\phi}^2$ along $\overrightarrow{ES}$ and a transverse component $(1/R)\ (d/dt)\ (R^2\dot{\phi})$ perpendicular to $\overrightarrow{ES}$, where (R, ϕ) are plane coordinates of S with origin at E.
The equation of motion in the radial and transverse direction are

$$m(\ddot{R} - R\dot{\phi}^2) = \frac{-\gamma M m}{R^2}, \tag{4}$$

$$m\left(\frac{1}{R}\right)\left(\frac{d}{dt}\right)(R^2\dot{\phi}) = 0. \tag{5}$$

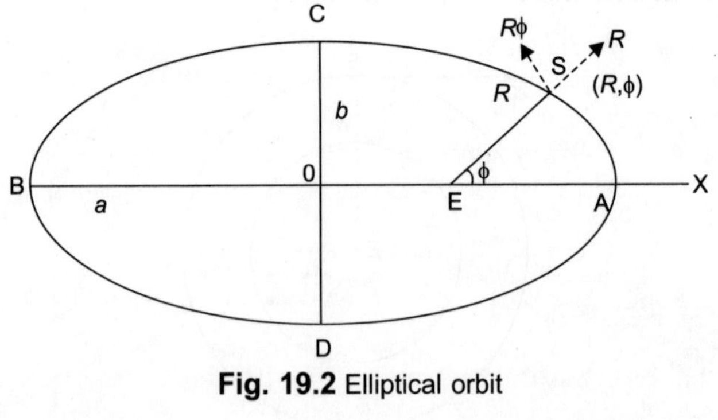

Fig. 19.2 Elliptical orbit

A first integral of (5) is

$$R^2\dot{\phi} = \frac{H}{m}, H \text{ is a constant.} \tag{6}$$

Here $R\dot{\phi}$ is the transverse component of the velocity of S, $mR\dot{\phi}$ is the transverse component of the momentum of S, while $R(mR\dot{\phi})$ is called the moment of this transverse component of momentum about the point E.

The radial component of momentum given by $m\,\dot{R}$ has no moment about E, as its line of action passes through E. Hence (6) means that the total moment of momentum of S about E is H; which is a constant. Geometrically (6) means that the rate of description of the sectorial area, $R^2(\dot{\phi}/2)$ by$\overline{ES}$ is constant and = $H/2m$.

19.3.5 Integration of the Equations of Motion

Energy equation: Substituting for $\dot{\phi}$ from (6) in (4), and integrating the resulting equations by multiplying both sides by $2\dot{R}$, we get $\dot{R}^2$. Using this value of $\dot{R}^2$; the total kinetic energy T of S is given by

$$T = \left(\frac{1}{2}\right) mv^2 = \frac{1}{2}m(\dot{R}^2 + R^2\dot{\phi}^2) = \left(\frac{Km}{R}\right) + E, \tag{7}$$

where E/m is a constant of integration in the first integral of (4) in terms of $\dot{R}^2$; and $K = \gamma M, -Km/R$ is called the potential energy V of S. The equation (7) is then called the energy conservation equation with total constant energy E:

$$T + V = E. \tag{8}$$

It gives the relation between v and R for a non-circular orbit (analogue of equation (1) for a circular orbit).

Orbit equation: By eliminating t from (4), (6), taking $u = 1/R$ and ϕ as the dependent and independent variables, and by measuring ϕ from a suitable initial radius vector $\overline{ES}$, one can integrate the resulting second order equation in u and ϕ to get

$$\left(\frac{H^2}{KM^2}\right) u = \frac{(H^2/KM^2)}{R} = 1 + \left(\frac{CH^2}{KM^2}\right) \cos\phi, \tag{9}$$

where C is an arbitrary constant depending on the initial condition. Comparing (9) with the standard equation of an ellipse in plane polar coordinates:

$$\frac{l}{R} = 1 + e\cos\phi, \tag{10}$$

we connect the physical constant in (9) with the geometrical constant l (semi-latus rectum) and e (the eccentricity) of the ellipse by

$$l = \frac{H^2}{KM^2}, e = \frac{CH^2}{KM^2}. \tag{11}$$

The initial conditions must be so chosen that $e < 1$.

Obvious connections with the other geometrical constants a (semi-major axis) and b (semi-minor axis) of the ellipse are now available with

$$l = \frac{b^2}{a}, \text{ and } b^2 = a^2(1 - e^2) \tag{12}$$

Using (7), the energy constant E can be shown to be

$$E = \left(\frac{-K^2 m^3}{2H^2}\right)(1 - e^2) \tag{13}$$

Then from (7), using the geometrical constants, one obtains:

$$v^2 = K\left(\frac{2}{R} - \frac{1}{a}\right) \tag{14}$$

which is the analogue of (1) for an elliptic orbit.

Period: Since (1/2) $(R^2\dot{\phi}) = H/2m$ (see equation (6)) is the rate of description of the sectorial area of the ellipse by the radius vector $\overrightarrow{\mathrm{ES}}$, the period, which is the time required to describe the total area $\pi\ ab$ of the ellipse, can be computed and expressed as

$$T^2 = \left(\frac{4\pi}{K}\right)a^3 \tag{15}$$

which is the analogue of (3) in conformity with Kepler's third law: The square of the period is directly proportional to the cube of the semi-major axis.

Apses and Apsidal distances: The points A and B in Fig. 19.2, where the velocity of S is perpendicular to $\overrightarrow{\mathrm{ES}}$ (the ends of the major axis) are called the apses. The nearest and furthest apses A and B are respectively called the perigee and apogee. Obviously $\dot{R} = 0$ at A and B and hence from (7), $R_1 = \mathrm{EA}$ and $R_1 = \mathrm{EB}$ can be shown as the roots of the apsidal equation

$$R^2 + \frac{Km}{E}R - \frac{H^2}{2mE} = 0$$

19.4 Some Important Problems in Satellite Dynamics

Using the theory explained in the preceding section, it is now possible to discuss some important problems in satellite dynamics.

19.4.1 Problems when the orbit is circular

The following aspects are important and may be of interest to the reader.

a. Velocity of S needed to reach a given height above the Earth's surface or vice versa.

b. Smooth tangential landing of the satellite on the Earth's surface.

c. Minimum number of satellites required to communicate a signal simultaneously throughout the Earth.

Velocity for a given height:

Equation (1) solves this problem directly. For example for $h = 100$ km, the rockets must give a velocity of 7.8 km/s to the satellite, if the values of γ, M, R_E RE are taken as in Section 19.3.

Height for a given velocity: This problem is particularly important when the number of revolutions of the satellite above the Earth's surface per day is prescribed in advance.

When the satellite is at rest relative to the Earth (rotates about E with the angular velocity ω of the Earth), the prescribed velocity is

$$v = (R_E + h)\omega \tag{17}$$

$$\text{where } \omega = \frac{2\pi}{24} \times 60 \times 60 \text{ radians/s} \tag{18}$$

Substituting the value of ω obtained from (17) in (18) and using the constants in Section 19.3, the required height h above the Earth's surface:

$$h \cong 35800 \text{ km} \tag{19}$$

This solution is important for a communication satellite, which must reflect signals to the same fixed receiving stations all the time.

If the satellite is required to be above a fixed station twice a day, its angular velocity ω_1 must satisfy

$$\omega_1 - \omega = \frac{4\pi}{24} \times 60 \times 60 \text{ radians/s}$$

where ω is the angular velocity of the Earth given by (18). Since $v = (R_E + H)\omega_1$ is the velocity of the satellite, h can be obtained from (1) as before.

Smooth tangential landing of S on the Earth's surface:

Here the direction of the velocity of S must be changed without a change in its magnitude. Suppose $h = R_E$ so that S is describing a circular orbit of radius $2R_E$ (Fig. 19.3). If its direction is changed through an angle α, its moment of momentum about E becomes

$$H = m(2R_E)\left(\frac{K}{2R_E}\right)^{1/2} \sin\left(\alpha + \frac{\pi}{2}\right) = m(2R_E K)^{1/2}\cos\alpha.$$

The point where S touches the Earth's surface will be required to be the closest apse (perigee) of the subsequent elliptic path of S, with $R_1 = R_E$. Hence from (6) and (3)

$$R_E^2 - 4R_E \cdot R_E + 4\cos^2\alpha R_E^2 = 0,$$

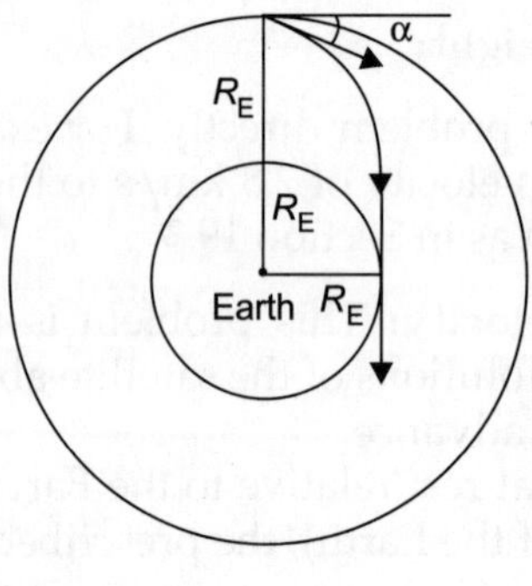

Fig. 19.3 Smooth return of a satellite

which gives $\alpha = 30°$.

Number of stationary satellites required to cover the Earth:

How many (minimum) satellites, all fixed relative to the Earth, will be required if, for example, a live cricket match is to be shown all over the world on a TV screen?

Since each satellite is fixed relative to the Earth, it describes a circular orbit of height 35800 kms (See equation (19)) above the Earth.

Any such satellite will cover an angle on the Earth's surface given by Fig. 19.4.

$$\cos\alpha = \frac{R_E}{h + R_E} = \frac{6368}{42140}.$$

Thus $\alpha \approx 81°$.

Hence at least three stationary satellites will be required to cover the entire Earth.

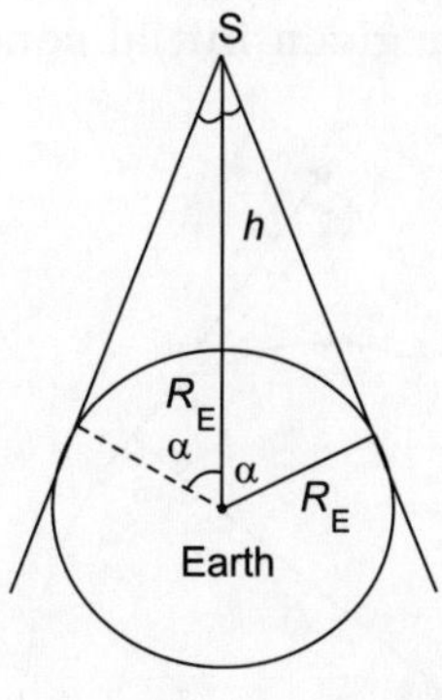

Fig. 19.4 Angle subtended by Earth at a stationary satellite

19.4.2 Problems when the orbit is elliptic

The following interesting problems will be briefly discussed.

a. Maximum and minimum velocities of the satellite for its given orbit.
b. Dependence of the geometrical constants of the orbit on its initial conditions.
c. Interception of one satellite by the other, when both are initially moving in the same orbit.
d. Satellite motion to hit a given point on the other half of the Earth. (ballistic trajectory).

These problems are now considered one by one.

Velocity limits for a given orbit

If a, e are the geometrical constants of the predesigned orbit, then

$$\text{Min } R = R_1 = EA = a(1-e),$$

while Max $R = R_2 = EB = a(l+e)$.

Hence from equation (14)

$$\frac{K}{a}\frac{1-e}{1+e} < v^2 \le \frac{K}{a}\frac{(1+e)}{(1-e)}.$$

Geometrical constants for given initial conditions

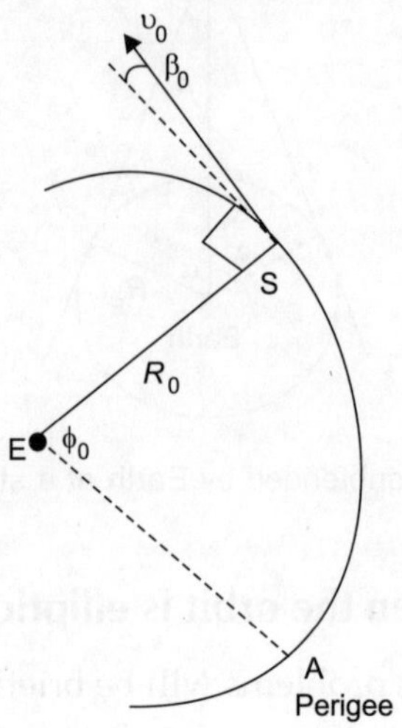

Fig. 19.5 Initial conditions for projection of S.

Suppose that when the fuel in the rocket carrying the satellite S is completely burnt out, ES $= R_0$, the initial velocity of S is v_0, and the direction of the velocity makes an angle β_0 with the normal to ES through S, $R_0\phi_0$ are the initial plane polar coordinates of S (Fig. 19.5). It is required to find the geometrical constants l and e of the elliptic orbit and $\phi_0 = \angle$SEA for given β_0, v_0, R_0, where A is the closest apse (perigee) of the orbit. If the initial point of projection of S is fixed, the corresponding perigee is located by ϕ_0 when l, e are computed.

The initial momentum at $t = 0$ (which remains constant subsequently) is

$$H = mRv_0 \cos\beta_0 \tag{20}$$

Substituting for H from (18) in equation (13), one obtains

$$e^2 = (1 + R_0 v_0^2/K)((R_0 v_0^2/K) - 2)\cos^2\beta_0 \tag{21}$$

Now from equation (11)

$$l = \left(\frac{R_0^2 v_0^2}{K}\right)\cos^2\beta_0 \tag{22}$$

so that,

$$\frac{l}{R_0} = \left(\frac{R_0 v_0^2}{K}\right)\cos^2\beta_0 \tag{23}$$

Substituting for l/R_0 and e from (23) and (21) respectively in (10), and re-arranging, one obtains:

$$\tan\phi_0 = \left(\frac{R_0 v_0^2}{K}\right)\frac{\cos^2\beta_0\sin\beta_0}{(R_0 v_0^2/K)\cos^2\beta_0 - 1}. \tag{24}$$

The dependence of e, l/R_0 and ϕ_0 on the heading angle β and the factor $R_0 v_0^2/k$ may be specially noted.

Interception of one satellite by another:

Two satellites S_1 and S_2 move initially in the same circular orbit of radius R_0 about the Earth, S_2 is leading S_1 by a specified angle ϕ_0; and S_1 is pursuing S_2. Now the direction of velocity of S_1 is changed so that subsequently it describes an elliptic orbit and catches S_2 at C as in Fig. 19.6

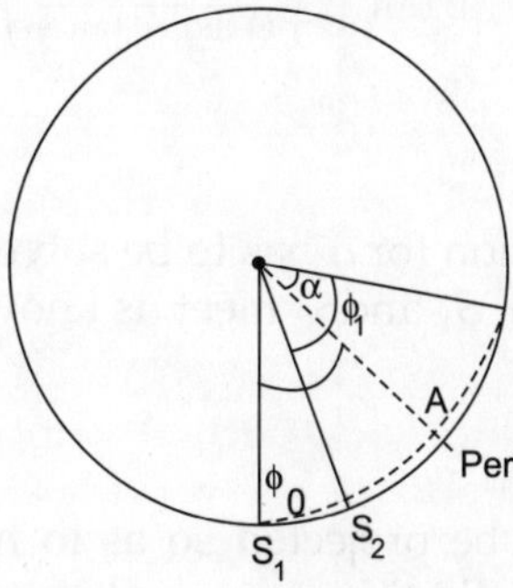

Fig. 19.6 Interception on a circular orbit

Let the $\angle$ S_2EC = ϕ_1. It is given that the new orbital arc S_1AC is symmetric about EA, so that A is the perigee of the new orbit. Then $\alpha = \angle AEC = (\phi_0 + \phi_1)/2$. The point C is thus determined when α is found out.

Let $(l/R) = 1 + e\cos\phi$ be the equation of the new elliptic path of S_1 along S_1AC. The angle α is determined using the fact that the time required by S_1 for the path S_1AC is the same as the time required by S_2 along the circular path S_2C. From equation (3), the time required by S_2 upto the position C

$$= \left(\frac{2\pi R_0^{3/2}}{K^{1/2}}\right)\left(\frac{\alpha}{2\pi}\right) = \alpha R_0^{3/2}K^{-1/2} \tag{25}$$

This is twice the time taken by S_1 from A to C.

Now, using (6), (11), (10), one obtains

$$\frac{dt}{d\phi} = \frac{a^{3/2}(1-e^2)^{3/2}}{K^{1/2}(1+e\cos\phi)^2} \tag{26}$$

Integration of (25) from 0 to α gives the required time by S_1 from A to S.

The technique of integration requires the use of

$$\left(\frac{d}{d\theta}\right)\left(\frac{e\sin\phi}{1+e\cos\phi}\right) = -\frac{(1-e^2)}{(1+e\cos\phi)^2} + \frac{1}{(1+e\cos\phi)} \tag{27}$$

where, as usual the integration of $1/(1+e\cos\phi)$ with respect to ϕ, requires the expression to be changed in terms of tan $(\phi/2)$. Hence, using (25), the final result after some calculation is

$$(1-e^2)^{3/2}a = (1+e\cos\alpha)^{3/2}\left[2\tan^{-1}\left\{\frac{(1-e)}{(1+e)^{1/2}\tan\frac{\alpha}{2}}\right\} - e(1-e)^{1/2}\frac{\sin\alpha}{(1+e\cos\alpha)}\right] \tag{28}$$

This transcendental equation for α has to be solved numerically for α, so that the position C, where, S_1 andS_2 meet, is known.

Ballistic Trajectories

A ballistic missile S is to be projected so as to hit a given target point T on the other half of the Earth's surface. It is required to i) determine the direction of projection for L, ii) to find the direction of projection for getting the maximum range on the Earth's surface and iii) to find the maximum height h of the missile S above the Earth's surface.

The initial conditions for this problem are $R = R_E, v = v_0, \beta = \beta_0$ at $\phi = \phi_0$, $t = 0$ (Fig. 19.7). The eccentricity e of the orbit corresponding to these initial conditions, obtained using equation (21), is

$$e^2 = 1 + \left(\frac{R_0 v_0^2}{K}\right)\left(\frac{R_E v_0^2}{K} - 2\right)\cos^2\beta_0 \tag{29}$$

From equation (24), since $\phi_0 + \alpha/2 = \pi$, one obtains

$$\frac{\tan\alpha}{2} = \frac{R_E v_0^2}{K}\frac{\sin\beta_0\cos\beta_0}{\left(1-\left(\frac{R_E v_0^2}{K}-2\right)\cos^2\beta_0\right)} \tag{30}$$

The angle α determined from this equation gives the range arc $LT = R_0\alpha$. Alternately if $R_0\alpha =$ LT and α is already known for the given target position T and launch position L; then equation (29) gives β_0, the angle of projection, after a numerical calculation.

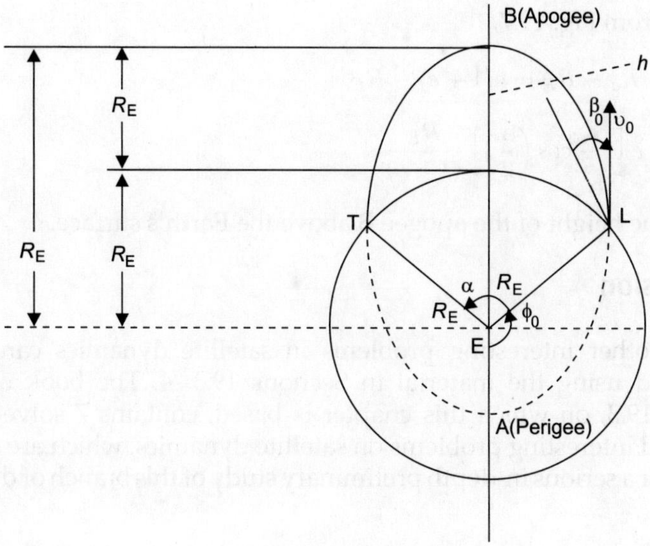

Fig. 19.7 Ballestic trajectory

Maximum possible range can be obtained by maximising α or $\tan \alpha/2$ as a function of β_0 in (28). The usual theory of maxima from differential calculus then gives the angle β_0 for which $\tan \alpha/2$ is maximum:

$$\sin^2 \beta_0 = \frac{1 - \left(\dfrac{R_E v_0^2}{K}\right)}{2 - \left(\dfrac{R_E v_0^2}{K}\right)} \tag{31}$$

The maximum angle is then obtained by substituting from (31) into (30):

$$\tan \frac{\alpha}{2} = \frac{\left(\dfrac{R_E v_0^2}{K}\right)}{2\left[1 - \left(\dfrac{R_E v_0^2}{K}\right)\right]^{1/2}}. \tag{32}$$

α given by (32) gives the maximum range $R_E \alpha$.

Since L has polar coordinates $(R_E, \pi - \alpha/2)$, using equation (10), (12), one obtains,

$$R_E = \frac{a(1-e)^2}{1 - e\cos(\alpha/2)}. \tag{33}$$

Hence, from Fig. 19.7,

$$h = R_a - R_E = a(1+e) - R_E$$

$$= e\left[1 - \cos\left(\frac{\alpha}{2}\right)\right]\frac{R_E}{(1-e)}. \tag{34}$$

This is the height of the apogee B above the Earth's surface.

Conclusion

Several other interesting problems in satellite dynamics can now be discussed using the material in Sections 19.3–4. The book quoted in Section 19.3, on which this chapter is based, contains 7 solved and 16 unsolved interesting problems on satellite dynamics; which are all worth trying for a serious in-depth preliminary study of this branch of dynamics.

Lecture 20

Rocket Flights

Abstract

In this lecture we will develop the mathematical theory of rocket flight and use it to determine the terminal speed of the rocket (and the load carried by it) at the time when all the fuel in the rocket is exhausted. It will also be shown how the speed can be further enhanced by using a two stage rocket with alternative optimal ratios of the masses of the two rockets (about 10:1)

20.1 Introduction

We are familiar with tiny rockets—we see them as crackers during Deepawali and other enjoyable moments. Such rockets on a large scale have gained great importance during the twentieth century due to two significant uses: i) They are used in wars for targeting enemy craft. ii) They are used in space technology for launching satellites, space stations or astronauts to the moon or in space. Rockets are thus the prerequisites for further space dynamics like those discussed in the previous lecture. The elementary mathematical principle behind rocket flights should therefore be studied by every mathematics lover.

20.2 Equation of Motion of a Rocket and its Solution

All of us are familiar with the shape of a rocket. Its upper portion called the pay load (which may be a satellite or a bomb etc.) is supported by the lower portion, which when ignited propels out mass through the lower end (Fig. 20.1). This gives a propulsive force to the rocket which moves in a direction opposite to the direction of motion of the propelled mass.

Let $m(t)$ be the mass of the rocket at time t. This mass consists of the mass of the rocket containing the remaining fuel at time t and the pay load P carried out by it.

The initial mass at $t = 0$ is $m(0) = m_0 + P$, where m_0 is the initial constant mass of the rocket excluding the pay load P, but including the entire fuel in it. Let $v(t), v + \delta v$ be the speeds of the rocket at time $t, t + \delta t$ respectively, while δm_p is the mass propelled out from the rocket during the time interval δt with a speed $u(t)$, subject to the condition that the speed of the propellant relative to the rocket:

$$v(t) - (-u(t)) = v + u = c = \text{constant.} \tag{1}$$

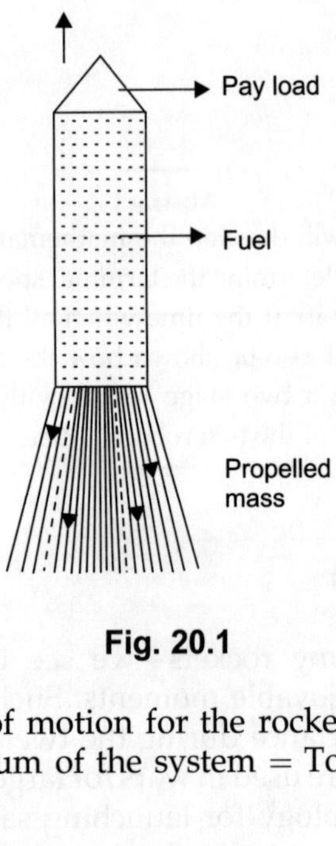

Fig. 20.1

Newton's equations of motion for the rocket–fuel system is: Rate of change of total momentum of the system = Total external force on the system.

Thus

$$\lim_{\delta t \to 0} = \left[\frac{\{m(t) - \delta m_p)(v + \delta v) + \delta m_p(-u)\} - mv}{\delta t} \right] = F$$

So

$$\frac{mdv}{dt} - (u + v)\frac{dm_p}{dt} = F \tag{2}$$

Using equation (1) and the fact that

$$\frac{dm_p}{dt} = -\frac{dm}{dt} = k = \text{constant.}$$

Equation (2) becomes,

$$m\frac{dv}{dt} + c\frac{dm}{dt} = -mg.$$

The force of gravity is extremely small in comparison with the propulsive force on the rocket due to mass ejection. Hence neglecting it in the first approximation, equation (4) can be written as

$$\frac{dv}{dm} = -\frac{c}{m}, \tag{5}$$

$$v = 0 \text{ for } m = m_0 + P \text{ at } t = 0. \tag{6}$$

The solution of (5), (6) gives the speed of the rocket at any time t:

$$v = -c \ln\left[\frac{m}{m_0 + P}\right]. \tag{7}$$

This is the addition to the initial zero speed with

$$m(t) = m_0 + P - kt \tag{8}$$

by (3).

Terminal maximum speed V:

This is obtained when all the fuel of total mass ϵm_0 (say) is exhausted and $m = m_0 - \epsilon m_0$

Then

$$V = -c \ln\left[\frac{1-\epsilon}{1+\beta}\right], \ \beta = \frac{P}{m_0}. \tag{9}$$

Here ϵ is the ratio of the fuel mass to the total initial rocket mass. For all practical purposes, its value is about 0.8, while β = ratio of pay load to initial total mass and is about $1/100$. Hence from (8), the terminal maximum speed is

$$V = 4.7 \text{ km/s}. \tag{10}$$

20.3 Additional Rocket for a Satellite Projection

We have seen in Lecture 19 on satellite dynamics that the minimum speed required to put a satellite in a circular orbit around the earth is about 7.8 km/s. Hence V given by (9) should be further increased. This can be done by using a two stage rocket.

Two stage rocket: At $t = 0$, the pay load P is supported by two portions of the rocket, the lowermost portion is filled with m_1 units of fuel, while the upper portion contains a mass m_2 units of fuel.

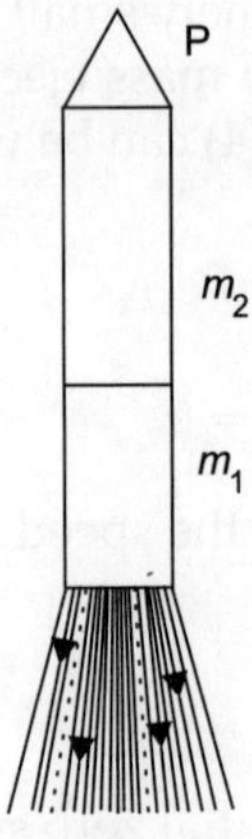

Fig. 20.2

The case of the first stage rocket (the lowest portion) is thrown off as soon as the fuel of mass m_1 in it is completely burnt out, giving a terminal speed,

$$V_1 = -c \ln \left[1 - \frac{\epsilon m_1}{m_1 + m_2 + P} \right]. \tag{11}$$

Equation (11) is obtained from (9) by replacing P with $m_2 + P$ and m_0 with m_1; which are now the pay load and initial mass excluding the pay load, respectively.

As soon as the first stage rocket is burnt and thrown off, the second stage rocket is ignited. It adds to (11) a speed of magnitude.

$$\overline{V} = -\epsilon \ln \left[1 - \frac{\epsilon m_2}{m_2 + P} \right] \tag{12}$$

Equation (12) is again obtained from (9) by taking

$$m_0 = m_2, \ P = P, \ \beta = \frac{P}{m_2}, \ \epsilon = \epsilon \tag{13}$$

Adding (11) and (13), the net terminal speed, V_2 of the pay load P, after both the rockets are burnt out, is,

$$V_2 = V_1 + \overline{V} = -c \ln\left[1 - \frac{\epsilon m_1}{m_1 + m_2 + P}\right]$$
$$-c \ln\left[1 - \frac{\epsilon m_2}{m_2 + P}\right] \tag{14}$$

It is required to get V_2 as large as possible by internal adjustments of the initial masses m_1 and m_2 of the two rockets such that the total initial mass of the rocket is a constant equal to m_0 say.

This is the problem of maximising V_2 in (14) subject to the constraint

$$m_1 + m_2 = m_0. \tag{15}$$

Using (15), V_2 in (14) can be expressed as a function of m_2 only and its maxima as a function of m_2 can be obtained from the theory of maxima in calculus of one real variable by using

$$\frac{dV_2}{dm_2} = 0 \text{ and } \frac{d^2V_2}{dm_2^2} < 0 \tag{16}$$

In this way it is found that V_2 attains its maximum value for

$$m_2 = -P + (P_2 + Pm_0)^{1/2}. \tag{17}$$

The corresponding value of m_1 is obtained from (15). The ratio of m_1 to m_2 for maximum V_2 turns out to be

$$\frac{m_1}{m_2} = \left(1 + \frac{1}{\beta}\right)^{1/2} \tag{18}$$

where $\beta = \dfrac{P}{m_0}$. (19)

Substituting for m_2 from (17) and then for m_1 from (15), the maximum possible speed V_2 is obtained from (14) for

$$m_1 = m_0(1+\beta)^{1/2}[(1+\beta)^{1/2} - \beta^{1/2}]; \tag{20}$$

$$m_2 = m_0[-\beta + (\beta + \beta^2)]^{1/2}. \tag{21}$$

The entire phenomenon is controlled only by three parameters; the initial total mass m_0 of the rocket, the pay load P to be carried out; and constant speed c of ejection of the propellant mass relative to the rocket.

Numerical data

In general, the normal data for rocket flight is

$$\epsilon = 0.8, \; c = 3 \text{ km/s}, \; \beta = \frac{1}{100}. \tag{22}$$

Then from (18),

$$\frac{m_1}{m_2} \approx 10.05. \tag{23}$$

The first stage rocket must be about 10 times heavier than the second stage rocket, if maximum speed is to be attained. Further, using (22) in (20), (21) and (14), the maximum possible speed turns out to be

$$V_2 = 7.65 \text{ km/s}. \tag{24}$$

This is slightly less than the speed of 7.8 km/s, but we are now close to the desired maximum speed for satellite projection in a circular orbit. By suitably altering the data, particularly c, we can reach the required speed of 7.8 km/s.

Another alternative is to use a third stage rocket, but then additional costs are involved. This may be unavoidable if a very high speed is required.

20.4 Further Studies

The development of the theory, technology and uses of a rocket has a long history of at least 700 years [2]. Nowadays a variety of solid or liquid fuels are used as propellants [2]. Nuclear core rockets have also been developed.

It can be shown that if external forces such as, air resistance and gravity are neglected, the terminal speed of the rocket is independent of the way in which the propellant is ejected, even if it varies with time [2]. Hence the model with constant c, considered here, is a good approximation for all practical purposes.

The problem of maximisation of the terminal speed with the help of multistage rockets (more than 2) can also be analysed on the lines of the theory for a two stage rocket. Let m_0 be the least total mass of the rocket excluding the pay load P required to get a terminal speed of 7.8 km/s. Then a graph of m_0/P (where m_0 is the least possible mass of the rocket including the fuel but excluding the pay load required to get a terminal speed of 7.8 km/s) against the number of rocket stages used, is given in Fig. 20.3.

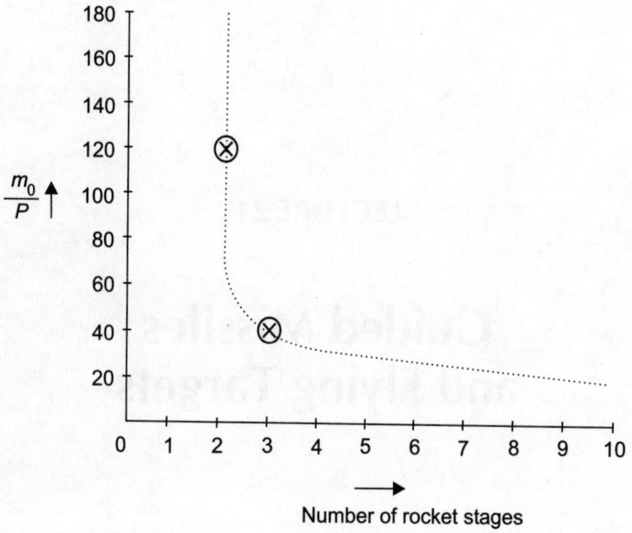

Fig. 20.3

The graph shows a considerable decrease in m_0 from stage 2 to stage 3. However, there is only a small decrease in m_0 from stage 3 to stage 4 and so on. Thus it is clear why NASA prefers a three stage rocket to other higher stage systems involving considerable further increase in the cost at the cost of a minor saving in the input minimum mass.

Conclusion

It is hoped that this elementary study of rocket flight within the scope of the graduate level mathematics, based on the two books: 1) Burghes D N and Borrie M S 's *Modelling with Differential Equations*, and 2) Burghes D N and Downs A M 's *Modern Introduction to Classical Mechanics and Control*, will initiate the readers to a further and deeper study of the more complex realistic problems of rocket dynamics.

LECTURE 21

Guided Missiles and Flying Targets

Abstract

A simple mathematical analysis of the pursuit of a target by a guided missile is presented here. The missile is fitted with a homing device by which the velocity of the missile is always directed towards the target. The time required by the missile to hit the target is computed. Thus the old topic of "pursuit curves" in classical mechanics has now acquired a renewed importance in the modern age of skud and missile wars.

21.1 Introduction

Guided missiles which can somehow sense the direction of the target have been talked about since ancient days. The Ramayana and the Mahabharata have cited many examples of weapons being destroyed by other weapons in mid-air. But in those days, guided missiles were just a concept, a visionary but powerful weapon of destruction. Now that concept has become a reality. Much of USA's victory in the Gulf War could be credited to their use of missiles fitted with a homing device against Iraqi skuds. These homing devices helped fix the direction of the velocity of the missile to be always in the direction of the target. Problems such as these which determine the ways and means of following or pursuing an object are known as pursuit curves in mechanics. A traditional version of it is the pursuit of a thief by a policeman, both running on a plain ground or a dog trying to catch a running cyclist.

21.2 Formulation of the Problem

The actual real problem of hitting a flying object is quite complicated. However, the problem can be introduced at the graduate level in its simplest form by avoiding the inherent complexities in the beginning. The intricacies can be gradually added to the problem subsequently by suitably modifying the initial simple problem.

Consider a target T moving in a horizontal straight line in air with a constant velocity of magnitude v_T. The starting point of the missile M is the origin O(0, 0) at $t = 0$. With y-axis along the vertical, and x-axis parallel to the path of T, let the coordinates of T at $t = 0$ be (a,b).

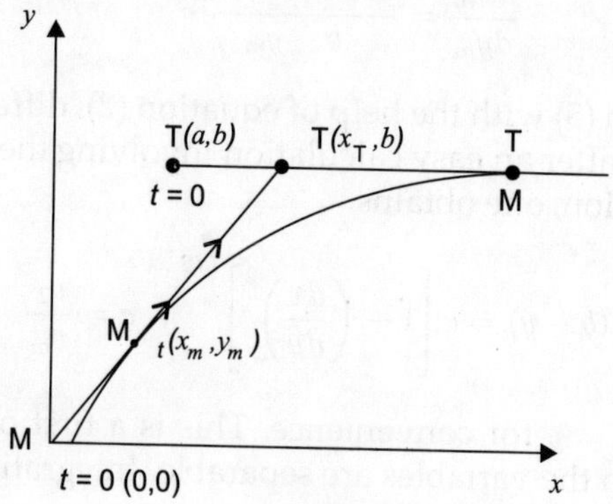

Fig. 21.1

At any time $t > 0$, M is at (x_m, y_m) while T is at (x_T, b); $\overrightarrow{MT}$ being the direction of velocity of M is tangential to the path of M. Ultimately, if M hits T, then the coordinates of M and T become equal at some time t_1. It is required to find t_1 and the position of M or T at t_1, i.e., to find when and where M hits T; given that the speed of M is a constant v_m.

21.3 Solution of the Problem

If the coordinates of T are (x_T, b) at time t, then

$$x_T = a + v_T t. \tag{1}$$

If M is at (x_m, y_m) at t, then the constant speed v_m of M is related to its component velocities by

$$\dot{x}_m^2 + \dot{y}_m^2 = v_m^2. \tag{2}$$

The direction of v_m is tangential to the path of M, and since the direction of velocity of M is along $\overrightarrow{MT}$ (guided missile),

$$\frac{\dot{y}_m}{\dot{x}_m} = \frac{b - y_m}{x_T - x_M}. \tag{3}$$

The initial conditions are

$$\text{at } t = 0, x_m = y_m = 0, x_T = a, t_T = b. \tag{4}$$

Equations (1) to (4) should be used to solve the problem.

21.3.1 Solution method

Equation (3) can be written, as

$$\frac{dx_m}{dy_m} = \frac{a + v_T t - x_m}{b - y_m} \tag{5}$$

To eliminate t from (5) with the help of equation (2), differentiate (5) with respect to t. Then, after an easy calculation involving the use of the chain rule of differentiation, one obtains,

$$\frac{d^2x}{dy^2}(b - y) = c\left[1 + \left(\frac{dx}{dy}\right)^2\right]^{1/2}, \quad c = \frac{v_T}{v_m} \tag{6}$$

where $x_m = x, y_m = y$ for convenience. This is a first order equation in $dx/dy = p$ in which the variables are separable. Integrating using,

$$p = \frac{dx}{dy} = a/b \text{ when } y = 0, \tag{7}$$

one obtains, dx/dy. A further integration using the initial conditions (5), yields,

$$x = \frac{1}{2}\left\{\frac{(b - y)^{(c+1)}}{(c+1)fb^c} \frac{fb^c(b - y)^{(1-c)}}{1 - c}\right\} + K_1. \tag{8}$$

where,

$$f = d + (1 + d^2)^{1/2}, \; d = a/b \tag{9}$$

and

$$K_1 = \frac{b|(f^2 + 1)c + f^2 - 1|}{2f(1 - c^2)}$$

The missile M hits the target T at time t_1 when the coordinates of T at time $t_1 : (a + v_T t_1, b)$ lie on the path (8) of M. This gives

$$t_1 = \frac{(a^2+b^2)^{1/2}+ac}{v_m(1-c^2)}, \tag{10}$$

which is the capture time at position $(a + v_T t_1, b)$.

The magnitude of the velocity v_m of M for a given capture time t_1 can also be determined from (10).

Conclusion

The problem, when the path of the target is a given plane (or three–dimensional) curve, not necessarily a straight line, can be studied using the above principles, but the mathematics is then not simple.

It has been demonstrated that the introduction of this important problem is possible at the graduate level using the mathematics taught at that level. A problem of this type is also solved in F Chorlten's *A Text Book of Dynamics* by using polar coordinates and taking $v_m = 2v_T$.

LECTURE 22

Mathematical Economics

Abstract

An introduction to this highly developed branch of economics is presented here particularly for students and teachers of science and engineering. It is shown that the consumer's demand and entrepreneurs supply to the market will match and an equlibrium state of the market, advantageous to all, can be attained, provided suitable optimisation polices, developed in this lecture, are followed by all.

22.1 Introduction

Mathematical economics is now a very well developed and useful branch of mathematics. Nobel's dictum of not giving a Nobel award to a mathematician has been over-ruled all because of the immense potential of mathematical economics to help humanity. Prof Scholes got it in 1997 and in 2001 Prof Amartya Sen, received a Nobel prize for his study of poverty based on mathematical and statistical analysis.

Since economics is generally taught by non-mathematicians in India, in the department of social sciences, while mathematics is prominently taught in the faculties of sciences and engineering, very few students study the theory of mathematical economics at the graduate level. Therefore a short elementary introduction to mathematical economics based on relevant portions from Ball, M A's *Mathematics in Social and Lifesciences*, parts SM and E, and Archibald, C G and Lipsey, R G's *A Mathematical Treatment of Economics*, is given here using graduate level mathematics.

22.2 Main Optimisation Problems

Any problem which involves getting maximum benefits in a given situation is called an *optimisation problem*. The following can be considered as an optimisation problem.

1. A consumer wants to get maximum satisfaction by spending as small an amount as possible on various items (commodities) required.

2. Those who take decisions about the production of these commodities by changing inputs into outputs (called entrepreneurs) aim at minimum production cost for a fixed production, or equivalently aim at maximum production at a fixed cost. At the same time

3. They want maximum profit in the market at given market prices over which they have no control (unless they are the only producers and suppliers of a commodity). The only thing that they can control is the supply to the market.

Consumer's demand based on the optimisation in 1) should ultimately match the supply based on the optimisation in 2) and 3). Then the market is said to be in an equilibrium state. Such a stable economy is most desirable and beneficial to all. However, when there is an imbalance between demand and supply in the market, the economic system is dynamic. A mathematical theory tries to avoid this imbalance between demand and supply by solving the optimisation problems 1) to 3) above.

22.3 Consumer's Optimisation

A consumer has a variety of requirements called commodities $Q_1, Q_2, \ldots Q_n$. Various grains and groceries is an example. By adjusting the quantities $q_1, \ldots, q_n$ of these items to be purchased within a specified budget in a given unit of time, maximum satisfaction, or equivalently, utility is sought by the consumer. Since utility U depends upon $q_1, q_2, \ldots, q_n$, we can say that U is a function of $q_1 \ldots q_n$; say,

$$\mathrm{U} = f(q_1, q_2, \ldots, q_n). \tag{1}$$

There may be a variety of n tuples $(q_1, \ldots q_n)$ for which *U is the same*. They are all said to be equivalent. A surface passing through all of them is known as an *indifference surface*. If only two commodities are considered, the indifference surface becomes an indifference curve (Fig. 22.1).
For any two points A and B on this curve, the consumer gets the same satisfaction U_0. A consumer's tendency is to increase U_0 within the restriction of the budget allocation.

If $p_1, p_2, p_3 \ldots, p_n$ are the market prices per unit of $q_i, \ldots, q_n$, the expenditure y_A of the consumer A is

$$p_1 q_1 + p_2 q_2 + \ldots + p_n q_n = y_A. \tag{2}$$

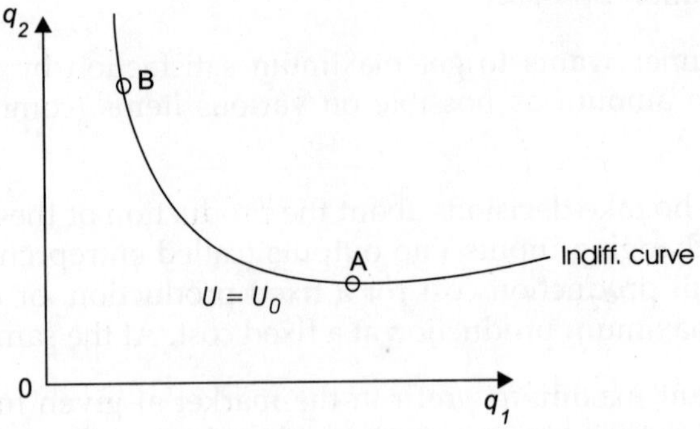

Fig. 22.1

Now if y_A is fixed by A and maximum U is required from (1), this is the problem of maximisation of the function $f(q_1, \ldots, q_n)$ in (1) subject to the constraint (2). This is a well formulated problem in mathematics.

For example, if f in (1) is a continuously differentiable function of $q_1, \ldots, q_n$, then the calculus of many variables gives the Lagrange multipliers method for solving this problem.

We shall not give the details of this well known method here, but then the outcome after using the method is that ultimately a set of values $(q_1^A, \ldots, q_n^A) = q^A$ of $q_1, \ldots, q_n$, all depending on $(p_1, p_2, \ldots p_n) = p$ are obtained for which U is greatest for A. In short, for obtaining the greatest possible value of U subject to the restriction (2),

$$q^A(p) = (q_1^A(p), \ldots, q_n^A(p)). \tag{3}$$

This $q^A(p)$ in (3) is called the demand function for the consumer A, for the price level p, which has n components $q_1^A, \ldots q_n^A$.

Example: Suppose a consumer's utility function for two items, say bread and milk, is given by

$$U = \frac{(q_1 + 6)(q_2 + 6)}{q - 1 + 2q_2 + 18} \tag{4}$$

where q_1, q_2 are respectively the units of bread and milk per month, while p_1, p_2 are respectively their prices for each unit. For a fixed monthly allocation y_0 of the budget, the price constraint is

$$q_1p_1 + q_2p_2 = y_A. \tag{5}$$

U in (4) should be maximised subject to the constraint (5). This problem can be solved using the theory of maxima and minima for two variables, using Lagrange multipliers.

The solution is,

$$q_1^A = \left(\frac{2}{p_1}\right)^{1/2} \frac{6p_2 + 6p_1 + y_A}{p_2^{1/2} + (2p_1)^{1/2}} - 6, \tag{6}$$

$$q_2^A = \left(\frac{2}{p_2}\right)^{1/2} \frac{6p_2 + 6p_1 + y_A}{p_2^{1/2} + (2p_1)^{1/2}} - 6. \tag{7}$$

Equations (6) and (7) determine the demand as a function of prices p_1, p_2 for maximum possible satisfaction of the consumer A. The quantities, q_1^A, q_2^A given by (6), (7) are the components of the demand function which may be denoted by $D(p, y_A)$.

In general for n commodities, the demand function is given by,

$$q_i^A = D_i^A(p, y_A), i = 1, 2, \ldots, n. \tag{8}$$

22.3.1 Consumer's Aggregate Demand Function

This is obtained by adding together the demand functions of all consumers over a period of time.

$$q(p) = \sum_A D^A(p, y_A)$$

$$= D(p, y_A, y_B, y_C, \ldots);$$

where $y_A, y_B, \ldots$ remain fixed over a period of time, thus

$$q = D(p) \tag{9}$$

is the demand function for a given price level p for the set of consumers A,B,C,. . ., over a period of time.

REMARK: It is neither possible nor necessary to measure the utility of A, which is an abstract concept. It is the indifference relation $f(q_1, q_2, \ldots, q_n) =$ constant that is important. The construction of this surface for a given consumer A requires statistical data over different periods of time and a smooth curve or surface fitting through this data.

22.4 Role of the Firm and the Entrepreneur

A firm is an input–output system which changes inputs such as raw material, labour, machines etc., (each one has its own costs) to an output called the product having a market price not controlled by the firm. Let us consider various firms producing the commodities $Q_1, Q_2, \ldots, Q_n$ as per the optimal aggregate demand of the consumers determined in the previous section. An *entrepreneur* is the decision maker in the firm who takes economic decisions related to inputs, production, supply to the market etc. This may be a single person or a group of persons or a computer etc., who has to consider two important problems.

1. Input–output levels and

2. Production cost.

The input–output levels are the rates of flow of quantities of inputs or outputs per unit time. This unit time will depend upon the type of production. It may be a year for agricultural outputs. But the unit of time should not be so large that there are changes in the mechanism of production called *technology*, which is not the concern of economics.

For simplicity, we consider only one of the n commodities, call it Q and denote the quantity of Q produced per unit time by q. Let $x_1, x_2, \ldots, x_n$ be the input levels. These are the quantities of the inputs $X_1, X_2, \ldots X_n$ per unit time. The output level q depends upon the input levels through a known relation

$$q = F(x_1, x_2, \ldots x_n). \tag{10}$$

called the *output function*. The set of all $x = (x_1, x_2, \ldots x_n)$ for which the production q is the same, determines a surface

$$F(x_1, x_2, \ldots, x_n) = q^0 \tag{11}$$

called the *isoquant*.

If $r_1, r_2, \ldots, r_n$ are the costs per unit of the inputs $X_1, \ldots, X_n$, with input levels $x_1, x_2, \ldots, x_n$, then the total cost $C(x)$ of production of q units of Q is given by

$$C(x) = b_0 + r_1x_1 + r_2x_2 + \ldots + r_nx_n. \tag{12}$$

Here b_0 is the fixed maintenance cost even if there is no input. The entrepreneur will either maximise the production function F in (10) for a fixed production cost $C = C_0$ in (12) or equivalently minimise the production cost C given by (12) for a fixed given production q^0 in (11).

This mathematical problem is similar to the problem of consumer optimisation considered in the previous section. Its solution gives the production cost C as a function of the production q or vice versa; say

$$C = C(q) \tag{13}$$

where C is the minimum production cost for the given production q.

22.4.1 Maximum Market Profit

Let p be the market price of a unit of production Q in the previous section. If the sale determined as per demand is q units, in a suitable unit of time, the revenue collected after the sale is

$$R = pq. \tag{14}$$

The profit of the firm is

$$\pi = pq - c(q). \tag{15}$$

This profit is maximum for a given market price p for those values of q for which $\pi'(q) = 0$ and $\pi''(q) < 0$.

That is, from (15),

$$p - C'(q) = 0, \tag{16}$$

and $$C''(q) > 0. \tag{17}$$

From (17) it is clear that the curve (Fig. 22.2)

$$y = C'(q) \tag{18}$$

is a strictly increasing curve. It intersects the curve

$$y = p = \text{constant} \tag{19}$$

in atmost one point. The unique point of intersection

$$q = q^0 = f(p) \tag{20}$$

is the solution of (16). The corresponding maximum profit given by (15):

$$\pi = q^0 \left(c'(q^0) - \frac{\pi(q^0) + b}{q^0} \right) \tag{21}$$

must be positive. Otherwise, if π is negative or zero, the firm should shut down production.

The relation (20) is one–one and is a strictly increasing function of p if the given market price p changes. Hence (16) is

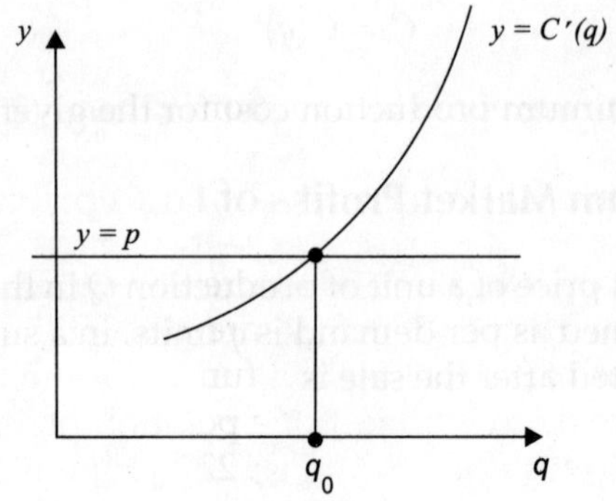

Fig. 22.2

one–one. Therefore the inverse function obtained from (16):

$$q = S_f(p) \tag{22}$$

for the firm is also monotone in p if p varies. This is called the *supply function* of the firm and controls the supply of the firm to the market. If there are many firms producing the same product Q, each one will optimise the production and profit, and will thus have its own supply function.

The aggregate supply function

$$S(p) = \sum_f S_f(p) \tag{23}$$

for various firms producing the same product controls the total supply to the market, when each firm tries to maximise the production at a fixed cost and maximise the profit at the given market price not controlled by the firm. This must match the aggregate consumer demand $D(p)$, equation (9), based on consumers' optimisation.

22.5 The Market Behaviour

A market is a set of conditions under which producers sell and consumers buy a certain commodity. If the number of commodities is more than 1, say $Q_1, Q_2, \ldots Q_n$, then it is called a multi-market. For simplicity we shall consider a market for a single commodity.

22.5.1 Market Equilibrium

This market, is said to be in equilibrium if there is no change of demand, supply, price etc. An essential requirement for equilibrium is that the demand from the consumer must match the supply from the firm.

$$D(p) = S(p) \tag{24}$$

where $D(p)$ and $S(p)$ are given by equations (9) and (23).

22.5.2 Existence and Uniqueness of Equilibrium

If the price increases, the demand decreases, while the supply from the firms increases. Hence $D(p), S(p)$ are respectively decreasing and increasing functions of p (Note that all functions and variables are non-negative). Therefore there is atmost one point of intersection $p = p_e > t_0$ of the curves $y = D(p)$ and $y = S(p)$ (Fig. 22.3); for which

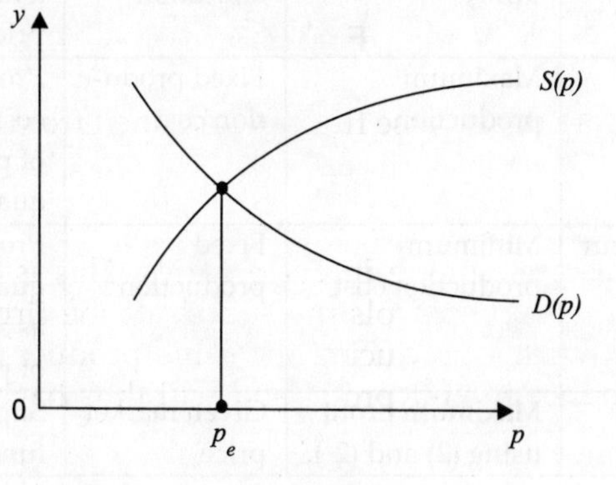

Fig. 22.3

$$D(p_e) = S(p_e) \tag{25}$$

The demand supply and price remains constant over a period of time.

The other theoretical possibilities, where $S(p)$ and $D(p)$ do not intersect (which do not generally occur in a practical situation), are shown in Figs. 22.4 and 22.5.

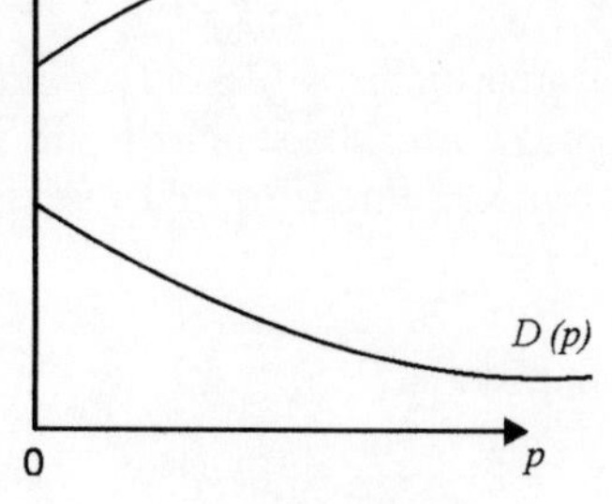

Fig. 22.4

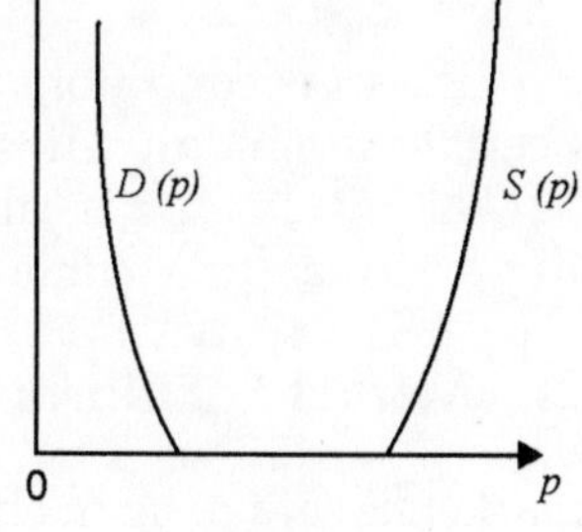

Fig. 22.5

In the situation given by Fig. 22.4, the commodity (such as air) is freely available; while for Fig. 22.5; the market settles at $D = S = 0$, in equilibrium.

Conclusion

In short, three main optimisation problems govern an economic system in a suitable unit of time.

System element	Objective	Constraint	Outcome
1) Consumer	Maximum utility	Budget allocation	Demand D as a function of price p: $D(p)$
2) Entrepreneur	Maximum production	Fixed produ-tion cost	Production cost as a function of produced quantities
2') Entrepreneur	Minimum production cost	Fixed production	Produced quantities as a function of production cost
3) Entrepreneur	Maximum profit using (2) and (2').	Given market price	Supply S as a function of price

A stable economy requires that $D(p) = S(p)$. Then if the total demand, production, supply and sale phenomenon is governed by the optimisation processes described here, the consumer, the producers, and the entrepreneur all get the best possible advantage of the total system. We hope that graduate students and their teachers, particularly in science and engineering, will be motivated by this simple mathematical analysis to study more complex real problems in mathematical economics faced by our country.

Bibliography and Additional Reading

Lecture 1
History of Fields Medals

1. Devi, Indu. The Fields Medals, *Science Today*, a publication of *Times of India*, Mumbai, India. pp 51–52, Jan 1979.

2. Monostyrsky, Michael. *Modern Mathematics in the Light of the Fields Medals*. Natick, MA: A. K. Peters. 1998.

3. Riehm, Carl. The early history of the Fields Medals, *Notices of AMS*, Vol. 49 (No. 7): 778–782. 2002.

4. Tropp, Henry S. The origin and history of the Fields Medals, *Historia Math* 3: 167–181. 1976.

Web Sites:

i. http://www.history.mcs.st-andrews.ac.uk/history/socities/fieldsmedals.html

ii. http://elib.zib.de/IMU/Medals/

iii. http://www.fields.utoronot.ca/aboutus/fieldsmedals-monastyrsky.pdf.

Lectures 2, 3 and 4
Chaos Before Cantor
Order Out of Chaos
Paradise Lost Paradise Regained

1. Richard, Courant and Robbins Herbert. *What is Mathematics*? 2nd Ed. Oxford University Press. 1996.

2. Davis, P J and R Hersh. *The Mathematical Experience*. London: Penguin. 1983.

3. Huzurbazar, V S. *What is Mathematics*? Mysore: Mysore University Publications. 1967.

4. Kline, Morris. *Mathematics in Western Culture.* New York: Oxford University Press. 1953.

5. Kline, Morris. *Mathematics, The loss of Certainty*. New York: Oxford University Press. 1986.

6. Russell, B. *Mysticism and Logic and other Essays*. Pelican Books. 1981.

7. Gamow, G. *One, Two, Three. . .Infinity: Facts and Speculations of Science.* New York: Dover Publications. 1988.

8. Kumbhojkar, H V. Myth of Sisyphus: Ism in mathematics. R C Gupta Endowment Lecture. Association of Mathematics Teachers of India (AMIT). 2001.

9. Vilenkin, N Ya. *Stories about Sets.* London: Academic Press. 1968.

Lecture 5
Concerns of a Mathematician

1. Boyer, Carl B. *A History of Mathematics.* 2nd Ed. Revised by Uta C Merzbach. New Jersey: John Wiley & Sons. 1991.

2. Dunham, William. *The Mathematical Universe: An Alphabetical Journey Through the Great Proofs, Problems and Personalities.* New Jersey: John Wiley & Sons. 1994 (Chapter on Justification).

3. Jhunjhunwala, Ashok. *Indian Mathematics: An Introduction*. New Delhi: Wiley Eastern. 1993.

4. Kashikar, P K. The Archimedian solids. *The Mathematics Students* 2 (No. 2): 60–65. 1934

5. Krishnamurthy, V. *Culture, Excitement and Relevance of Mathematics.* New Delhi: Wiley Eastern. 1990.

6. Lakshmikantham, V and Leela. *The Origins of Mathematics.* Oxford: University Press of America, Inc. 2000.

7. Newman, James R. *The World of Mathematics.* 4 volumes. New York: Simon and Schuster. 1956.

8. Singal, Asha Rani. Mathematics: An unexpected pleasure. *The Mathematics Student* 65 (No. 1–4): 1–35. 1996.

9. Steward, Ian. *The Magical Maze.* London: Wiedenfeld & Nicolson. 13–15. 1997.

Lecture 6
Friendly and Changing Ways of Teaching Mathematics

1. Balachandra Rao, S. *Indian Mathematics and Astronomy: Some Landmarks.* 2nd Ed. Bangalore: Jnana Deepa Publications. 2000.
2. Bhatnagar, P L. *Introductory Lessons on Modern Mathematical Concepts.* New Delhi: Affiliated East West Press. 1971.
3. Datta B and A N Singh. *History of Hindu Mathematics,* (Two volume set edition). New Delhi: Bhartiya Kala Prakashan. 2001.
4. Deo, S G and Howell, G W. A highway to trigonometry. *Bulletin of the Marathwada Mathematical Society* 1: 26–62. Dec. 2000.
5. Guy, R K and Woodrow (ed.).*The Lighter Side of Mathematics.* Washington, DC: The Mathematical Assocation of America. 1994.
6. Krishnamurthy, V. Right way to teach maths. *The Hindu,* May 22. 1990.
7. Rao, A R. *A Manual of Mathematical Models and Teaching Aids.* Ahmedabad: Vikram Sarabhai Community Science Centre. 1993.
8. Summers, George J. *The Great Book of Puzzles and Teasers.* Mumbai: Jaico Publishing House. 1996.
9. Tikekar, V G. Chemical anologies in mathematics teaching. *Bulletin of the Marathwada Mathematical Society* 1: 134–136. 2000.

Lecture 7
Coping With Reality

1. Klir G J and B Yuan. *Fuzzy Sets and Fuzzy Logic: Theory and Applications.* India: Prentice-Hall, India. 1997.
2. Kosko, B. *Fuzzy Thinking.* Verlag: Flamingo. 1994.
3. Kumbhojkar, H V. Coping with reality with Fuzzy sets. Mathematics Newsletter, 7 (No. 3). 60–66. 1997.
4. Kumbhojkar, H V. Arresting imprecision by mathematics. *Proc. of the 26th Annual Iranian Mathematics Conference* 193–199. 1995.

Lecture 8
Conjectures in Mathematics

1. Dunham, William. *The Mathematical Universe: An Alphabetical Journey Through the Great Proofs, Problems and Personalities.* New Jersey: John Wiley and Sons. 1994. Chapters on " Euler ", and on " Prime Number Theorem ".

2. Ganitanand. Some mathematical lapses from Aryabhata to Ramanujan. *Ganita Bharati (Bulletin of Indian Society for History of Mathematics* 18 (1996): 31–47.

3. Gardner Martin, *The 2nd Scientific American Book of Mathematical Puzzles and Diversions*. New York: Simon & Achuster. 1961.

4. Guy, Richard. *Unsolved Problems in Number Theory*. 3rd ed. New York: Springer. 2004.

5. Gupta, H R. Partitions – An introductory survey. in *Ramanujan---An Inspiration*, edited by P K Srinivasan, Madras. 1967.

6. Hasse, H and Prichatt G D. The determination of all four-digit Kaprekar constants. *J. Reine Angeas. Math.* 299/300 (1978): 113–124.

7. Hoffman Paul. The man who loves only numbers. *The Atlantic Monthly*. Nov. 1987.

8. *Mathematics Teacher* (India) [Official Journal of the AMTI – Association of Mathematics Teaches of India (B19, Vijay Avenue, 37, V R Pillai Street, Triplicane, Chennai 600005)], Special Felicitation Issue on D R Kaprekar.

9. Mihailescu, P. Primary, cyclotomic units and a proof of Catalan's conjecture. *J. Reine Angew. Math* (Gelle's Journal) 572 (July, 2004,): 167–195.

10. Yogananda, C S. Fermat's last theorem – A theorem at last! *Samasya*, 5 [(Nos 1 to 3), May & Sept (1998) and Jan (1999)]: 35–41.

Lecture 9

How Well We Learn and Teach Mathematics

1. Albers D J. (Ed.) *Mathematical People: Profiles and Interviews*. Basel: Birkhauser. 1985.

2. Hardy, G H. *A Mathematician's Apology*. Cambridge: Cambridge University Press (1940). 1967.

3. Hildebranat Stefan, and Anthony Tromba. *Mathematics and Optional Form*. New York: W. H. Freeman & Co. 1985.

4. Kapur, J N *Fascinating World of Mathematical Science*, Vols. 1–8, Mathematical Sciences Trust Society (1989–90).

5. Kline, Morris. *Mathematical Thought from Ancient to Modern Times*. New York: Oxford U. Press. 1972.

6. Krishnamurty, V. The culture of mathematics teaching. *The Mathematics Students*, 65 (Nos 1 to 4): 110–116. 1996

7. Singh, P K. Glimpses of the development of mechanics from Ancient Period to Renaissance. *Ganit Bharati*, 24: 25–34. 2002.

8. Rao, A R. *Brain Sharpeners*. Vikram A. Sarabhai Community Science Centre. 1995.

Lecture 10
Primes and Composites

1. Das Gupta, S. The story of prime number. *Ganita Bharati*. 16 (Nos 1 to 4): 37–52. 1994.

2. Dunham, William. *The Mathematical Universe: An Alphabetical Journey through the Great Proofs, Problems, and Personalities*. New Jersey: John Wiley & Son. 1994.

3. Hoffman, Paul. *Archimedes' Revenge: The Joys and Perils of Mathematics* (Part I, Chapter 3). New York: Fawcett Columbine. 1988.

4. Honsberger, Ross. The generation of prime numbers (Chap 4). in *Mathematical Gems II (The Dolciani Mathematical Expositions, No. 2)*. The Mathematical Association of America. 1976.

5. Kanigel, Robert. *The Man Who Knew Infinity: A life of the Genius Ramanujan*. Maxwell MacMillan International. 1991.

6. Kapur, J N. Fascinating prime numbers. *Indian Journal of Mathematical Education, II* [(3), Oct (1991)]: 111–118.

7. Singh, Simon. *Fermat's Enigma*. New York: Walker Pub. Inc. 1997.

8. Srinivasan, P K. (Ed.) *Ramanujan, an Inspiration*, Madras. 1967.

9. Vaidya, A M. The variety of techniques in classical number theory. *The Mathematics Students*, 65 (Nos 1–4): 224–231. 1996.

Lecture 11.
Story of Multi-Story Numbers

1. Deo, S G. The story of multistorey-number system. *Junior Mathematician*. Association of Math. Teachers of India. 17–24. 1992.

2. Hall, H S and S R Knight. *Higher Algebra*. First published by Macmillian and Company Ltd (1887). Reprinted by S Chand and Company Ltd.,New Delhi. 1994. 557.

3. Hardikar, T B. *Indeterminate Analysis, Ancient and Modern*. Pune: P T Hardikar. 1991.

Lecture 12
Festival of Triangles

1. Andrews, G E. A note on partitions and triangles with integer sides *AMM* 477–478. 1979.
2. Bender, E A. Area perimeter relations for two-dimensional lattices. *AMM* 69: 742–744. 1982.
3. Dickson, L E. *History of the Theory of Numbers*. (1919–1923). New York: Chelsea reprint. 1952.
4. Fine, N J. On perfect triangles. *AMM* 63: 3–44. 1956.
5. Gould, H W. A triangle with integral sides and area. *Fibonacci Quarterly* 27–39. Feb. 1973.
6. Hammer, J. On a general area parameter relation for two dimensional lattices. *AMM* 71: 534–535. 1986.
7. Jordan, J H, Walch Ray and R J Wisner. Triangles with integer sides. *AMM* 98 (199): 686–689. 1995.
8. Krier, Nicholas and Benner Manvel. Counting integer triangles, *Math. Magazine* 71 (No. 4). 291–295. 1988.
9. Pepls, R R. Perfect triangles. *AMM* 62. 365. 1955.
10. Scott, P R. An area and parameter problem. *AMM* 81. 884–885. 1974.
11. Subbarao, M V. Perfect triangles. *AMM* (April, 1971): 384–385.
12. Whiteworth, W A and D Biddle in L E Dickson's *History of the Theory of Numbers* Vol. II. pp. 199. New York: Chelsea. 1952.

Lecture 13
Correction of Incorrectly Transmitted messages

1. Liu, C L. *Elements of Discrete Mathematics*. Second edition. New York: Mc.Graw Hill. pp. 347–384, 1986.
2. Trembley, J P and R Manohar. *Discrete Mathematical Structures with Applications to Computer Science*. New York: Mc.Graw Hill. 343–363. 1984.

Lecture 14
On Distance

1. Deo, S G. What is distance? *Ganit Shikshan*, 47. March 1995.
2. Euler, Russell and Jawad Sadek. The π go full circle. *Mathematics Magazine* 72, (3) Feb. (1999).

3. Hamming, R W. Error detecting and error correcting codes. *Bell System Tech. Journal* 29: 147–460. 1950.

4. Krause, Eugene K. *Taxicab Geometry: An Adventure in Non-Euclidean Geometry*. New York, NY: Dover Publications, Inc. 1986.

5. Rhodes, Frank. A geometric duality metrics in the plane. *Mathematical Gazette*. 54: 19–23. 1970.

6. Schattschneider, Doris J. The taxicab group. *American Mathematics Monthly* 91 (7): 423–428. 1984.

Lecture 15
Modeling with Differential Equations

1. Burghes, D N and M S Borrie. *Modelling with Differential Equations.* West Sussex: Ellis Horwood Ltd. 1982.

2. Braun, Martin, C S Coleman and D A Drene. *Differential Equation Models*. New York: Springer. 1982.

3. Henssge, Claus, Bernard Knight, Thomas Krompeclher, Burkhard Madea and Leonard Nokes. *Estimation of the Time since Death in the Early Postmortem Period*. New York: Hodder Arnold Publication. 1994.

4. Shendge, G R. Modelling with differential equations. *Bulletin of the Marathwada Math. Soci*. 1: 122–131. Dec. 2000.

Lecture 16 and 17
A Highway to Trigonometry I & II

1. Bushaw, D. Functions defined by differential equations. A Short Course in Trigonometry. *College. Math. Journal*. Volume 2: 32–35. 1971.

2. Deo, S G, V Lakshmikantham and V Raghavendra. *A. Textbook for Ordinary Differential Equations,* 2nd Edition. New Delhi: Tata McGraw-Hill. 1998.

3. Deo, S G and G Howell. A highway to trigonometry. *Bull of Marathwada Math. Soc.* 1: 26–62. 2000.

4. Joshi, S R and G R Shendge. A note on hyperbolic functions. *The Mathematics Students* XLIII, 1: 55–57. 1975.

5. Mikusinsksi I G, Sur Les Functions

$$K_n(z) = \sum_{v=0}^{\infty} (-1)^n \frac{z^{n+kv}}{(n+kv)!}, \quad k = 1, 2 \ldots, \quad n = 0, 1, \ldots, k-1$$

Ann Soc. Pon. Math. 21, 46–51. 1948.

6. Nagy, B. Approximation theorems, for cosine operator functions. *Acta Math. Hungarica* 69–76. 1977.

7. Nagy, B. On cosine operator functions in Banach space. *Acta Sci. Math.* 36: 281–290. 1974.

8. Pethe, S P and A Sharma. Functions analogous to completely convex functions. *Rocky Mountain J. Math.* 3: 591–617.

9. Richmond, D E. Trigonometry from differential equations. *Amer. Math. Monthly*, 61: 337–340. 1954.

10. Travis, C C and G G Webb. Cosine families and abstract nonlinear second order differential equations. *Acta. Math. Acad. Sci. Hung.* V. 32: 75–96. 1978.

Lecture 18

Mathematical Theory of Collective Decisions

1. Taylor, Michael. The problem of salience in the theory of collective decision making. in *Mathematical Approaches to Politics*, edited by H R Alker et al. Amsterdam: Elsevier Scientific Publishing Co. 231–255. 1973.

Lecture 19

Satellite Dynamics

1. Burges, D N and A M Downs. *Modern Introduction to Classical Mechanics and Control*. West Sussex: Ellis Horwood Ltd. 1975. Chapter 7, 146–185.

2. Kasture, D Y. Satellite dynamics. *Bulletin of the Marathwada Math. Soc.* 3: 75–86. 2002.

Lecture 20

Rocket Flights

1. Burghes, D N and M S Borrie. *Modelling with Differential Equations*. West Sussex: Ellis Horwood. 1982.

2. Burghes, D N and A M Downs. *Modern Introduction to Classical Mechanics and Control*. West Sussex: Ellis Horwood Ltd. 1975.

Lecture 21
Guided Missiles and Flying Targets

1. Burghes, D S and M S Borrie. *Modelling with Differential Equations.* West Sussex: Ellis Harwood. 1982.

2. Chorlton F. *A Text Book of Dynamics.* New Delhi: CBS Publlishers. 1990.

Lecture 22
Mathematical Economics

1. Archibald, C C and R G Lipsey. *A Mathematical Treatment of Economics.* Third Edition. London: Weidenfeld and Nicolson. 1980.

2. Ball, M A. *Mathematics in the Social and Life Sciences: Theories, Models and Methods.* Parts SM and E. West Sussex: Ellis Horwood. 1985.

3. Kasture, D Y. Mathematical economics. *Bulletin of the Marathwada Math. Soc.* 5(1). 2004.

Index